WHY ARE YOU STILL DIZZY?

UNDERSTANDING VESTIBULAR MIGRAINE

a long story about the dizziness business

ALEV ÜNERI, MD

To Cüneyd, Ali, and Ayşe,

This book is dedicated to you with all my love and gratitude. Thank you for your persistent patience (which I know can be quite a task sometimes), unwavering understanding (even when it may be exhausting), and boundless inspiration. You have been my rock, source of motivation, and support. I cherish each moment spent with you and am endlessly grateful for your presence.

ACKNOWLEDGEMENTS

I am deeply grateful to Prof. Dr. Necmettin Pamir, founder and president of the Marmara University Neurological Sciences Institute, for giving me the invaluable opportunity to work and conduct research there. Additionally, I want to extend my heartfelt thanks to my assistant Ayfer Kücükmetin, for her unwavering support, hard work, and cherished companionship throughout these years.

TABLE OF CONTENTS

INTRODUCTION

Why Are You Still Dizzy?

When I sought guidance from a friend's literary agent regarding my book on vertigo, the response was disheartening yet reflective of a sobering reality: "What's the point? Thousands of vertigo books are out there, and everybody who had vertigo I know is still dizzy." It was a poignant moment, one that underscored the magnitude of the challenge ahead and sparked a crucial question: Why is "everybody who had 'vertigo' still dizzy?"

That was already my driving force to write the book: Why, despite seeking help and receiving a diagnosis, do people continue to experience dizziness?

After dedicating most of my professional career to patients grappling with vertigo, dizziness, and imbalance and spending countless hours listening to their struggles with the debilitating effects, I knew—despite the abundance of existing literature—there is more to be said on the matter, driving me to turn a deaf ear to discouragement and instead, I decided to continue to write.

The most common disorder you've never heard of...

While burrowing the world of vertigo for further research, I uncovered stories of patients transcending the boundaries of fame and success. These were narratives not of red-carpet events or championship victories but of individuals facing a relentless adversary: vertigo.

Among them, Laura Hillenbrand, celebrated for her literary prowess with works like *Seabiscuit* and *Unbroken*, shares her struggle: 'I have vertigo. Vertigo makes it feel like the floor is pitching up and down. Things seem to be spinning. It's like standing on the deck of a ship in really high seas.' [1] Jason Day, a former top-ranked professional golfer, echoes this sentiment: "So hopefully I won't have another episode here. It's vertigo. It comes and goes. There is a concern at the back of my mind, but I just have to deal with that and go out and play golf. It happened at the US Open, and I'm just hoping it doesn't happen again here." [2] Esha Gupta, a renowned Bollywood actress, adds her voice: "I have been battling vertigo for a long time. It's something that I deal with on a daily basis." [3]

By shedding light on the experiences of these well-known figures, their candid accounts underscore the reality that vertigo spares no one, regardless of status or achievement. These stories serve as a sad reminder that behind the glitz and glamour lie individuals grappling with profound health challenges. Through their struggles, we witness the disruptive power of vertigo on personal and professional lives, emphasizing the urgent need for understanding and support.

If you got it, all these stars have another thing in common with their "vertigo": They are still struggling with it. I am sure they sought and got help; their physicians must have given them treatments and therapies, but we understand from their expressions that they are still dizzy, continually or from time to time.

---

1 https://www.beliefnet.com/wellness/health/health-support/illness-and-recovery/what-price-glory.aspx

2 https://www.theguardian.com/sport/2015/jul/12/jason-days-vertigo-comes-and-goes-but-hes-confident-he-can-challenge-for-open

3 https://timesofindia.indiatimes.com/entertainment/hindi/bollywood/news/esha-gupta-battles-vertigo/articleshow/14387433.cms

As I pointed out, their narratives highlight the common enemy as "vertigo." But what if I tell you that "vertigo" is not a disease on its own but a symptom of an underlying disorder? In fact, the word "vertigo" is just a synonym for "dizziness," "giddiness," "wooziness," and many more similar names trying to describe the sensation. When you use the word "vertigo," you only say "I'm dizzy" in a different language, which is ancient Greek.

While I can't confirm the specific diagnoses of these stars, I speculate that (again, from their expressions) they may be experiencing Vestibular Migraine (VM). How can I make such a bold claim without personally examining them? Given that, after decades dedicated to treating thousands of patients with all kinds of "vertigo," I've come to believe that one of the most commonly overlooked disorders in medicine is VM, which causes chronic or repetitive bouts of dizziness (vertigo) until you recognize and treat it appropriately.

Despite its prevalence, the term "vestibular migraine" remains unfamiliar to many, even those grappling with its debilitating effects. Thus, this book is my attempt to share insights and experiences backed by scientific research, aiming to bridge the understanding of what VM is and how to manage it. It's a guide for health professionals to recognize what they might be missing in the underdiagnosis of VM, and to empower patients with VM to lead healthier lives.

Decoding Dizziness: Unveiling the Truth Behind Your Diagnosis

Listen to your patient, he is telling you the diagnosis.
– William Osler

Vertigo and dizziness are the world's second-most common health complaint, following pain. It is estimated that 15% to 35% of the general population will experience vertigo or dizziness at some point, with prevalence potentially even higher depending on the study criteria, as indicated by extensive population-based studies.[4-5] For instance, a 2009 epidemiological study estimated that about 35% of adults aged 40 years or older in the United States—approximately 69 million Americans—have experienced peripheral vestibular dysfunction as vertigo/dizziness[6] Additionally, in 2016, the National Institute on Deafness and Other Communication Disorders (NIDCD) reported that more than 1 in 20 children between the ages of 3 and 17—nearly 3.3 million—face similar issues. Altogether, research suggests approximately 80 million cases of peripheral vertigo in the United States alone in 2016.[7]

Many of these patients receive diagnoses from healthcare professionals for common diagnoses like Meniere's disease, benign paroxysmal positional vertigo (BPPV), chronic dizziness (CD), vestibular neuritis (VN; viral vertigo), or similar disorders. However, after years of practicing medicine and working with dizzy patients, I believe some diagnoses may not accurately capture the underlying issue. They may, in fact, be disguises for something else.

How do I know? Well, I'm not just a doctor treating vertigo and dizziness—I'm also a patient. In the 1990s, I experienced my first scotoma (migraine aura). Although I never experienced a migraine headache in my life, not even after that experience, I knew it was a kind of migraine occurrence. Nevertheless, a few years later, I had my first vertigo episode.

Through my experience treating thousands of patients and grappling with my condition, I've become keenly aware of the deep connection between vertigo and migraines. I'm convinced that many peripheral vertigo syndromes with different names are, in fact, linked to migraines.

4 Agrawal Y, Carey JP, Della Santina CC, Schubert MC, Minor LB. Disorders of balance and vestibular function in US adults. *Arch Intern Med.* 2009;169(10): 938-944.

5 Hülse, Roland; Biesdorf, Andreas; Hörmann, Karl; Stuck, Boris; Erhart, Michael; Hülse, Manfred; Wenzel, Angela. Peripheral Vestibular Disorders: An Epidemiologic Survey in 70 Million Individuals. *Otology & Neurotology.* 40(1): 88-95, January 2019. | DOI: 10.1097/MAO.0000000000002013.

6Newman, Toker DE, Hsieh YH, Camargo CA Jr, Pelletier AJ, Butchy GT, Edlow JA. The Spectrum of dizziness visits to US emergency departments: a cross-sectional analysis from a nationally representative sample. *Mayo Clin Proc.* 2008; 83:765–75.

7 Jahn K. Langhagen, T.Schroeder, A.S.Heinen F. Vertigo and dizziness in childhood–update on diagnosis and treat ment. Neuropediatrics. 2011 Aug; 42: 129-134

In my practice, I've observed a myriad of clinical features associated with conditions like Meniere's disease, BPPV, chronic dizziness, phobic postural vertigo, bilateral vestibulopathy, vestibular paroxysmia, and more—all of which, in some way or another, are related to migraines. Remarkably, the association between migraines and vertigo has been recognized for almost two millennia, though it was largely forgotten until recent decades when it was named vestibular migraine (VM).

Of course, I wasn't alone in recognizing VM as the primary culprit behind many reputed diagnoses. If one delves into the medical literature, numerous articles highlight the association of migraine with other common peripheral vertigo diagnoses. This trend emerged in the 19th century and has increased exponentially in the last two decades.

Predictably, the medical community is still cautiously approaching the issue, step by step. While VM is now recognized as a condition, there are still stringent criteria, often requiring the presence of a typical migraine headache, to secure a VM diagnosis. However, migraine is a complex condition, with a headache being just one of its potential features, if present at all. Unfortunately, few healthcare professionals are aware of the various clinical disguises of vestibular migraine; instead, they often view them as distinct clinical entities. Despite the numerous and sometimes bizarre manifestations of migraine beyond headaches, relying solely on this historical component (headache) for diagnosis may hinder healthcare professionals from making the most informed decisions for their patients.

Another obstacle is the realization that simply labeling a condition as VM doesn't solve the problem for VM patients. While awareness of VM has gradually increased, the diagnosis is often added alongside other conventional diagnoses, treating it as a separate entity.

Undoubtedly, accurate diagnosis is a cornerstone of effective medical practice. Identifying VM as a form of migraine can profoundly alter the approach to treating vertigo patients. While the exact pathophysiology of migraines remains elusive, our understanding of managing them has evolved over two millennia.

Furthermore, undiagnosed VM not only deprives patients of appropriate treatment but also turns VM into a chronic, debilitating condition, significantly impairing their quality of life and imposing a substantial economic burden on both individuals and society.[8] Conversely, misdiagnosing VM as another condition, such as Meniere's disease, can lead to unnecessary surgeries and destructive or ineffective treatments, resulting in debilitating outcomes. Ironically, benign conditions like benign paroxysmal positional vertigo (BPPV), although typically responsive to the Canalith Repositioning Maneuver (CRM), still present challenges, with recurrence and persistent symptoms in some patients remaining unexplained. Recognizing the possibility of VM could address these issues and facilitate the path towards a healthier life for affected individuals.

Having spent decades treating dizzy patients, I am convinced that VM is one of the most commonly undiagnosed or underdiagnosed disorders. While academic writing must adhere to stringent scientific standards, clinicians often find that their experiences and observations provide invaluable insights beyond what academic publishing offers.

Inspired by works like Oliver Sacks' *Migraine*, which explores the intricacies of migraines, I embarked on a mission to share my knowledge and raise awareness about VM. My goal is to provide a comprehensive understanding of VM, encompassing its history, associated conditions like BPPV and Meniere's disease, treatment options, personal experiences, patient anecdotes, and self-care strategies for those living with VM.

However, it's important to clarify that VM is not the sole cause of peripheral vertigo and dizziness; numerous other conditions exist, ranging from easily detectable middle-ear infections to more complex issues like superior canal dehiscence syndrome. Nonetheless, after ruling out central nervous system-related causes, healthcare providers should consider vestibular migraine as one of the most common underlying causes for peripheral vertigo and dizziness.

---

8 Ruthberg J.S., Chandruganesh R., Armine K., Mowry S.E., Ottesson T.D. The economic burden of vertigo and dizziness in the United States. Journal of vestibular research, 01/2021, Volume 31, Issue 2 DOI:10.3233/VES-201531.

CHAPTER 1

NO, VERTIGO
IS NOT A DISEASE!

If a health professional diagnoses your dizziness as "vertigo," it's time to run—and run fast! While I might be adding a touch of drama, the truth remains: "vertigo" isn't a diagnosis with any real meaning. Allow me to illustrate. If you visit a doctor with pain and they diagnose you with "pain," you would rightly find it pointless, wouldn't you? Pain is merely a symptom of an underlying issue; for instance, knee pain may indicate a meniscus tear, which is a valid diagnosis. The same principle applies to vertigo. If you're experiencing dizziness (giddiness, wooziness, spinning of the head, whatever name you use to describe the sensation you are feeling) and your doctor labels it as "vertigo," your diagnosis is essentially meaningless.

In essence, vertigo isn't a disease. It's merely a symptom, often stemming from an issue within the vestibular system. Patients should be well-informed about their condition. If you're grappling with this "disorder," it's essential to educate yourself about the underlying problem you're facing.

What Does It Mean to Say "I'm Dizzy"?

We do not see things as they are, we see them as we are.
–Anais Nin

Do you remember the dizzying childhood games, like spinning around or playing the baseball bat spin? While feeling dizzy in those activities was like innocent fun, they can have a very different impact on individuals grappling with vertigo. If an adult were to attempt these spinning games, it would be much more challenging than for a child (children are closer to the ground and more flexible, making them less prone to serious injury while playing.) Now, imagine a perfectly healthy adult trying the dizzying bat game. Depending on the condition of their vestibular system, just a few spins might be enough to cause disorientation, or they might need several more spins. Shortly after stopping, standing becomes a challenge, and stumbling or falling is almost inevitable. This disorienting sensation is called vertigo.

This spinning sensation is accompanied by involuntary eye movements (nystagmus,) which create the illusion that the surroundings are in motion, which can be fascinating and unsettling. If the vertigo is intense enough, it may also lead to feelings of nausea.

Once the spinning sensation subsides, individuals may feel a vague sense of being unwell or disoriented, commonly called dizziness. In the medical world, dizziness typically refers to a milder form of vertigo. I tried a simplified explanation of vertigo/dizziness for those fortunate never to have experienced it firsthand.

As you can imagine, terms like vertigo, dizziness, and other similar phrases such as heavy-headedness, lightheadedness, giddiness, wooziness, wobbliness, and unsteadiness are the descriptors used by individuals experiencing vertigo. These adjectives attempt to convey a subjective sensation of movement even though no actual motion occurs.

Many of us have likely experienced some form of illusory motion at least once. However, because it's a purely subjective sensation, we each have our own impressions and ways of describing it. Those fortunate enough to be healthy often forget about the sensations they felt on a rollercoaster ride or similar experiences from years ago. Describing vertigo to someone who has never experienced it can be challenging, leading to fundamental communication issues between patients and physicians. Not-so-fun fact: I rarely struggled to ask the right questions in my practice and often surprised my patients with my precision. The secret? As a patient myself, I always understood the nuisance firsthand.

As a symptom of an underlying disease, the sensation of motion illusion (vertigo, dizziness) can vary significantly from one individual to another and from one episode to another. Some may perceive it as an accurate rotational movement of themselves or their surroundings, while others may experience it as a sharp, instant spinning sensation or a feeling of heaviness or wobbliness. Some even describe it as a soft swaying movement, akin to turning their head and seeing the scenery follow with a slight delay, which can be quite disturbing.

When these vertigo episodes are particularly intense, standing upright may become impossible, and keeping one's eyes open can be both challenging and irritating. This sensation of motion illusion results from a reflex movement of the eyes known as nystagmus, which we will explore further in the upcoming chapters.

Vertigo episodes can vary in duration, lasting only a few seconds or persisting for days, weeks, months, or even years. In prolonged cases, the vertigo may remain consistent, but it often waxes and wanes in intensity. When the episode subsides, patients may experience temporary relief and return to their previous state of health; although, unfortunately, recurrence is common. For some patients, however, the intense spell evolves into another common format of vertigo: chronic vertigo/dizziness, which presents one of the most challenging problems in medical practice.

In some cases, the chronic form of vertigo may manifest insidiously, with patients never experiencing a severe spinning vertigo episode. Instead, they may perceive a mild form of vertigo/dizziness, which persists steadily or fluctuates over time. In this manifestation of the disorder, the sensation is not a distinct movement but rather a continuous feeling of being heavy-headed, reminiscent of a hangover or drunkenness. Rapid head movements can exacerbate the sensation, leading to a perception of the surroundings slipping and potentially causing imbalance.

Vertigo in Childhood

It might surprise you, but vertigo and dizziness aren't exclusive to adults; children may be affected with vertigo/dizziness as early as toddlers. According to a 2016 report by the National Institute on Deafness and Other Communication Disorders (NIDCD), more than 1 in 20 children between the ages of 3 and 17—approximately 3.3 million children—have been diagnosed with dizziness or balance problems. This groundbreaking study, published in the *Journal of Pediatrics* by Ming-Li C. et al.,[9] represents the first large-scale, nationally representative survey of such issues in U.S. children, revealing that these problems are slightly more prevalent in girls and non-Hispanic white children.

The vestibular system is critical in developing normal motor control, postural adjustment, balance, and vision in children. Any disruption in this system can significantly affect a child's development. Unfortunately, vestibular problems in children are often overlooked, partly because young children, particularly toddlers, may not be able to articulate their symptoms effectively, and they may not fully comprehend the concept of vertigo or dizziness.[10]

As we understand, the vestibular organs provide crucial sensory information about motion and spatial orientation. By age six, both vestibular organs should function symmetrically, sending balanced signals to the

---

9 Jahn K. Langhagen, 2011

10 Jahn K. Langhagen, T. Schroeder, A.S. Heinen F. Vertigo and dizziness in childhood–update on diagnosis and treatment. *Neuropediatrics.* 2011 Aug; 42: 129-134

Alev Uneri

brain. However, vestibular issues in early childhood can impede the normal development of balance skills.[11]

Among children, mild vertigo is a common symptom. Head movements can trigger it, often leading to issues with visual precision, especially when turning to look at something. Nausea typically follows when the motion becomes provocative enough. Nystagmus, an involuntary eye movement, is another common symptom that vigilant parents can easily observe. Children with BPV may also exhibit sensitivity to motion (motion sickness), light, and sound, with symptoms typically subsiding after a period of sleep.

In medical circles, there's a penchant for classifications, leading to the recognition of a "specific" vestibular disorder in childhood known as childhood paroxysmal vertigo (CPV), also referred to as benign paroxysmal vertigo (BPV). BPV emerges as the most prevalent pediatric vestibular disorder, with a high likelihood that it's merely a migraine equivalent.

The ability to read in moving vehicles can be a reliable indicator for diagnosing motion sickness, especially in childhood. In adults, the response to the question "Do you have motion sickness?" can often be misleading due to adaptation. If your patient (or yourself) claims not to experience motion sickness, it's worth asking about their childhood experiences. Adaptation likely occurs when a susceptible individual gradually becomes asymptomatic with motion over time after experiencing numerous conflicting sensory events. In a 2014 research study involving over 800 children aged 7 to 12, 40% reported experiencing motion sickness when traveling by car or bus.[12]

By the way, who first described motion sickness? Indeed, it was none other than Hippocrates, who wrote: "Sailing on the sea proves that motion disorders the body."

---

11 Marcelli V. Piazza F. Pisani F. Marciano E. Neuro-otological features of benign paroxysmal vertigo and benign paroxysmal positioning vertigo in children: a follow-up study. *Brain & Dev.* 2006 Mar; 28: 80-84.

12 I.F. Henriques, D.W. Douglas de Oliveira, F. Oliveira-Ferreira., Motion sickness prevalence in school children., *Eur J Pediatr.* 173 (2014), pp. 1473-1482

An intriguing aspect of passive motion is that despite its provoking effect of motion sickness, it also has a calming effect. For instance, it's common to calm babies by rocking them gently, and even in adults, hugging a dear friend or someone you haven't seen in a while often involves rocking each other from side to side, a practice observed in most cultures.

In one paragraph, Oliver Sacks[13] summarized motion sickness perfectly: "Gentle passive motion is normally soothing and soporific—hence a baby may be rocked to sleep. In a certain portion of the population, however, the response to the passive motion (or direct vestibular stimulation) is excessive and intolerable—such people may suffer from intense "motion-sickness" in childhood (with nausea, vomiting, pallor, cold sweating, etc.) or after that; if a vascular headache is present in addition to the above symptoms, a motion migraine will result. Exaggerated responses to vestibular stimulation are perhaps the most common. Certainly, one of the most incapacitating idiosyncrasies of many migraine patients, and as such, they may be shut off from many of the simpler pleasures in life: swings in childhood, roller-coasters in adolescence, and traveling by bus, train, ship, or plane at all times. It is important to note that passivity and passive stimulation are essential in these reactions; many patients who are extravagantly prone to motion-sickness are perfectly able to drive their cars or pilot their boats and planes."

Did the term "motion migraine" catch your eye?

Planes, Trains, and Automobiles (and Boats Too!)

In the 1987 classic movie "Planes, Trains, and Automobiles," Del exclaims, "Next time, let's go first class, alright?" Yet, even the luxury of first-class travel can't shield you from the unpleasant grip of motion sickness.

You only need an intact vestibular apparatus and enough provocative stimulation to experience motion sickness. This provocative stimulation can

---

13 Sacks, O. (1995). Migraine, p. 117. Picador

take the form of physical motion, visual motion, or virtual motion. For example, if you are in a moving vehicle, whether it's a spaceship or a horse-drawn carriage (yes, even riding a horse can induce motion sickness), this constitutes physical motion. Watching fast-moving scenes, such as war scenes in the movie "Avatar" in an IMAX, is an example of visual motion. And if you're at Universal Studios, playing quidditch in "Hogwarts" and feeling queasy, this is an example of virtual motion.

Furthermore, in a recent study, researchers showed that patients with migraine responded to the visual stimuli differently compared to migraine-free participants, and they concluded: "Migraine is related to abnormal modulation of visual motion stimuli within brain regions, and these abnormalities relate to migraine disability and motion sickness susceptibility."[14]

The etiology and precise neurobiological mechanisms of motion sickness are ambiguous, and among the several hypotheses that have been proposed, the sensory conflict hypothesis is the most widely accepted theory; therefore, I can offer you only this one hypothesis on motion sickness; it is the "sensory conflict" hypothesis. I don't have anything more grounded than that, sorry, but it is a good one! It goes like this: When actual and expected motion don't overlap, motion sickness arises; that's it! Let's create an example to understand it better; imagine you are sitting in a cruise ship's restaurant on a stormy day. Now, while your proprioceptive system is trying to persuade you that you are sitting in a luxury restaurant chair, your vestibular system will tell another, possibly alarming story: the ship is rocking! If you are one of us (I mean, who has an overreacting vestibular system), you would be barfing already. Not funny!), or you may be an astronaut with a well-trained vestibular system, so you might continue to enjoy your delicious dinner; how inappropriate for pitiful us, while we are struggling with our autonomic reactions. These autonomic reactions include nausea, vomiting, pallor, sweating, hypersalivation, stomach awareness, and sleepy syndrome, referring to drowsiness, lethargy, and persistent fatigue. Elegant,

14 Carvalho G.F., Mehnert J., Basedau H., Luedtke K., May A., Brain Processing of Visual Self-Motion Stimuli in Patients with Migraine. An fMRI Study. *Neurology.* ep 2021, 97 (10).

yes...? No, of course not, I know, but Dramamine and its lethargic sleep or retching, no other options, the bell of the ball of the ship (you) should wait for the calm waters.

The issue at hand revolves around significant individual differences in motion sickness susceptibility within the population. This variability is believed to stem from gene–environment interaction, although it's not yet certain. More notably, a rather insidious form of motion sickness exists that you may not be familiar with. Graybiel and Knepton[15] were the pioneering researchers who first identified and described "sopite syndrome" as a symptom complex characterized mainly by drowsiness and lethargy and associated with motion sickness. The list of symptoms linked to sopite syndrome will pique your interest! The name is derived from the Latin word "sopite," meaning to calm or send to sleep. It differs from other manifestations of motion sickness and can occur independently, preceding other symptoms or in their absence. What's more concerning is that sopite syndrome may persist even after adapting to other symptoms of motion sickness. Yawning (potential behavioral marker), drowsiness, lethargy, apathy, decreased ability to concentrate, daydreaming, melancholy, boredom, disinterest, disinclination for work, mood changes, irritability, sleep disturbances, frequent daytime napping, mild depression, failure of initiative, and (very understandably) a desire to be left alone.

Twenty years later, this description gained credibility by ISO 5805, in which sopite syndrome was defined as "inordinate sleepiness, lassitude or drowsy inattention induced by vibration, low-frequency oscillatory motion (e.g., ship motion) or general travel stress."

Depending on the stimulus type, duration, and personal differences, sopite syndrome may be the only manifestation of motion sickness. Soporific symptoms usually appear before nausea and tend to remain after the cessation of the motion stimulus.

---

15 Graybiel A, Knepton J . Sopite syndrome: A sometimes sole manifestation of motion sickness. *Aviat Space Environ Med.* 1976; 47: 873 – 82.

Alev Uneri

If nausea follows soporific symptoms, then the diagnosis of motion sickness is obvious. However, sopite syndrome may be the main and only manifestation of motion sickness, making diagnosis extremely hard. Finally, the cherry on top is that sopite syndrome can persist for hours or even days, and if the exposure is prolonged, it can stay even longer.

Why Does Motion Sickness Matter?

I often received negative responses when I asked my patients about motion sickness. If I were to ask you now, you might respond the same: "Nope, I don't have motion sickness!" Most people answer this way, echoing the responses of my patients. But let me ask you differently: What was it like when you were a kid? Could you read a book in the back seat while your parents drove from, let's say, North Carolina to Illinois? How about seasickness? Did a boat ride in choppy waters ever make you feel queasy? Not even a touch of sopite syndrome?

Diagnosing whether you're susceptible to motion sickness is crucial because it can be related to migraines, and thus to your vertigo (see Chapter 8).

Before wrapping up this section, I must mention the fascinating "mal de debarquement" syndrome (MDD), which is a rare and poorly understood disorder of the vestibular system that manifests as a phantom sensation of self-motion, often described as rocking, bobbing, or swaying. Interestingly, I've experienced it several times after rocky boat trips. While they didn't last long, I welcomed them with a professional interest. Let me describe one incident: it was a windy day, and the sea was choppy; we spent the whole day on a boat, anchoring only three times briefly for swimming. Upon returning to shore late afternoon, I stepped onto land and experienced something shocking; the coastline seemed to rock as if I were still on the boat. It lasted a few hours after disembarking, and I found it amusing. However, many individuals who have experienced MDD likely didn't find it amusing, especially if they had no idea what was happening.

Is it intriguing and astonishing, even somewhat philosophical, to consider how we navigate our lives with such dependence and confidence on our sensory inputs, which are susceptible to deception?

Back to the professional realm: Most water-based activities, like ocean cruising, long-haul airplane travel, and even sleeping on waterbeds (odd, but it counts as a water-based activity in an extended stretch), may trigger mal de debarquement.

MDD symptoms tend to arise when you're not in motion, such as when lying down or standing still. While it's known that even healthy individuals may experience MDD after prolonged periods of passive motion, it typically lasts for seconds to three days. However, significant balance impairment can sometimes persist for months to years. Symptoms may diminish over time but can reappear spontaneously or after another exposure.

One More Bunny from the Hat: Phonophobia

Imagine your significant other attempting to help by hastily emptying the clean dishwasher, perhaps early in the morning. Plates and utensils clatter, clang, jingle, and bong. That sensation! It's disconcerting, like someone slapping your brain with a cymbal! You envision your partner as a blacksmith in rural Europe during the Middle Ages, using your brain as an anvil! If you can relate and find yourself contemplating getting rid of your partner, congratulations; you have phonophobia. Actually, the "phobia" part should technically belong to the other party, not to you, under these conditions, but let's not get into technicalities.

Nevertheless, the main takeaway (aside from not harming your significant other) is recognizing that you have a very low Loudness Discomfort Level (LDL). Intolerance to loud sounds often indicates the onset of hyperacusis, a clinical condition characterized by sensitivity to sound levels that are typically tolerable. Hyperacusis can stem from various diseases or health issues.

While migraine (drum rolls) and Meniere's disease have long been recognized as culprits of LDL, recent scientific literature [16] has shed light on phonophobia[17] and other auditory manifestations in vestibular migraine (VM).

16 Shi S., Wang T., Ren D., Wang W. Auditory Manifestations of Vestibular Migraine. *Front. Neurol.*, 15 July 2022 Sec. Neuro-Otology, Volume 13, 2022.

17 Dieterich M, Obermann M, Celebisoy N. Vestibular migraine: the most frequent entity of episodic vertigo. *J Neurol.* 2016 Apr; 263 Suppl 1:S82-9. doi: 10.1007/s00415-015-7905-2. Epub 2016 Apr 15.

CHAPTER 2

FROM ANCIENT WISDOM TO MODERN INSIGHT: HISTORY OF UNRAVELING THE INNER EAR

Human beings, who are almost unique in having the ability
to learn from the experience of others, are also remarkable
for their apparent disinclination to do so.
–Douglas Adams

Carl Sagan said,[18] "You have to know the past to understand the present."
It would be reasonable to add "and to imagine the future." It may sound
fanciful, but imagining and planning the future based on our memories
of the past is a neural mechanism that we use repeatedly in our everyday
life. Furthermore, research shows that we use much of the same neural

---

18 Sagan, S. (2011). *Cosmos* (p. 62). Ballantine Books.

Alev Uneri

machinery to both imagine the future and remember the past.[19] We usually aren't aware that we're looking at the future through a lens of the past, of course, but if we stop and think for a moment, it seems almost obvious how impossible it is to imagine and create a future without the benefit of memories of past experience. Science and technology are no different in this respect. Every new discovery, every exciting innovation is born from the discoveries and innovations that preceded it. Sometimes we have to look back before we can begin to look forward.

This chapter is dedicated (in all senses of the word) to the past and all the great minds who have contributed to the current body of information about vertigo and the function of the inner ear. Space does not allow for a comprehensive discussion of all the work and contributions that have been made in this field across the centuries—I can offer only a snapshot—so I encourage you to take note of these names and investigate them further at your leisure.

Note: The observant reader will notice that the great minds discussed in this chapter are all male (although I do mention Phoebe Hearst), white, and, with the exception of Ibn Sina (Avicenna), who was Persian, Westerners. An historic and social analysis of that is outside the scope of this book, but let me just say that this is another area in which we can shape the future for the better by learning from the past.

Discovery of the Inner Ear, the Hidden Gem

The written history of medicine can be traced back to the Ancient Egyptians. In fact, given what appears in that written history, it seems to me that most modern medical knowledge and practices can be traced back to the Ancient Egyptians.

---

19 Schacter, D. L., Addis, D. R., & Buckner, R. L. (2007). Remembering the past to imagine the future: The prospective brain. *Nature Reviews Neuroscience*. 8(9), 657-661. https://doi.org/10.1038/nrn2213.

Much of what we know about the Ancient Egyptians' scientific knowledge can be found in four well-known medical papyri: the Ebers Papyrus, Hearst Papyrus, Berlin Papyrus, and Edwin Smith Papyrus. We don't know who wrote these papyri, but we do know that three of them are named after great minds who helped make past knowledge available to contemporary researchers: Edwin Smith, an American Egyptologist; Georg Ebers, a German Egyptologist; and Phoebe Hearst, an American philanthropist and suffragist (feminist). The Berlin Papyrus deviates from the others in that it isn't named after Heinrich Brugsch, the German Egyptologist who discovered—although technically, I guess, he rediscovered it, of course—and published it.

It's thought that the papyri were written around 1550 BC and that some of the information in them dates as far back as 3400 BC. Much has been written about these papyri, but one of my favorite observations about them comes from the researcher Joseph E. Hawkins. He wrote that "the few Egyptian medical papyri that have survived the ages suggest that there may have been some physicians of that era who dealt only with the ears, just as others had limited their practice to the eyes."[20] Apparently "over-specialization" among medical professionals was also a problem back then.

Ear diseases and treatments are discussed in the Edwin Smith Surgical Papyrus,[21] which is dated between 3000 BC and 2500 BC and is generally acknowledged to be the earliest known scientific document in existence. This papyrus contains details about battle injuries to temporal bones (bones located on both sides of the skull, behind the auricles, that consist of the external ear canals and contents of our middle and inner ears), and how those injuries affected the hearing and speech of the wounded. The

20 Hawkins, J. E. (2004). Sketches of otohistory part 1: Otoprehistory: How it all began. *Audiology and Neuro-otology* 9(2), 66-71. doi: 10.1159/000075997.

21 Feldman, R. P., & Goodrich, J. T. (1999). The Edwin Smith Surgical Papyrus. *Child's Nervous System.* 15, 281-284. https://doi.org/10.1007/s003810050395.

Ebers Papyrus,[22] from about 1500 BC, has a chapter titled "Medicines for the Ear with Weak Hearing."

The Edwin Smith Papyrus is the oldest known surgical document on trauma, and it looks like a military surgery manual. It contains detailed descriptions of the surgery of wounded ears, including how to clean, stitch, and dress them. The Ebers Papyrus is less comprehensive and contains only information about remedies and treatments for ear problems.[23]

None of these papyri contain an anatomical description of the inner ear. The world would have to wait until the second century AD. But I'm getting ahead of myself.

The next key figure in our story is the Greek philosopher Aristotle. He believed that there was a resonant space in the ear (not the inner ear!) or head that was filled with purified air and vibrated in response to sound, thus facilitating hearing. His theory remained unchallenged until the 18th century, when the Italian physician Cotugno[24] discovered that the inner ear is filled with fluid. But now I'm really getting ahead of myself!

Back to ancient Greece and Hippocrates of Kos (c. 460 BC–c. 370 BC), one of the most outstanding figures in the history of medicine. Even though Hippocrates did not add anything to the body of knowledge about the anatomy of the inner ear or the concept of vertigo per se, I believe he and his work are worth mentioning because of his overall contribution to the field of medicine. His methods were almost entirely empirical; he was a vigilant physician, and he had faithful disciples who wrote down every-thing he said and kept it for posterity (what a blessing!). Although he had only slight knowledge of ear anatomy, he was interested in ear infections

22 Stiefel, M., Shaner, A., & Schaefer, S. D. (2006). The Edwin Smith Papyrus: The birth of analytical thinking in medicine and otolaryngology. *Laryngoscope.* 116(2), 182-188. doi: 10.1097/01. mlg.0000191461.08542.a3.

23 Mudry, A. (2006, September 11–16). Otology in medical papyri in Ancient Egypt [Paper presentation]. Fifth Congress of the European Federation of OtoRhino-Laryngology Head and Neck Surgery, Rhodos/Kos, Greece. https://www.advancedotology.org/content/files/sayilar/59/buyuk/ Mudry.pdf.

24 Manni, E., & Petrosini, L. (2009). Domenico Cotugno (1736–1822). *Journal of Neurology* 257(1), 152-153. DOI:10.1007/s00415-009-5369-y.

and the ears' relationship to other organs.[25] In that respect, he took something of a holistic approach to his work.

That brings us to the second century AD. This was a defining period in its own way, as it's when the Greek physician-anatomist Galen described and named the inner ear. He chose to call it "labyrinth." Given the curving passageways of the inner ear, it is reasonable to assume he was inspired by the mythical Labyrinth, supposedly built by Daedalus for King Minos of Crete at Knossos. Although Galen may have had only slightly better knowledge of the anatomy of the ear than Hippocrates, his rules for the treatment of diseases including otitis, hearing loss, and tinnitus were followed to the letter for the next fourteen centuries. Yes, you read that correctly: "fourteen centuries." The American researcher Joseph Hawkins wrote of the post-Galen world, "Little if anything of value or significance was added to medical knowledge after the fall of Rome. In that sterile period, Byzantine physicians upheld, but did not expand, traditional Greek medical knowledge."[26]

However, not everyone was content to simply coast along during the post-Galen period. Persia's Ibn Sina (generally known as Avicenna in Western circles) (980–1037) took the stage in the 11th century and became one of the best-known physicians of his time.[27] As a polymath living in the middle of the Islamic Golden Age, Ibn Sina worked in the fields of medicine, philosophy, and astronomy, but he is probably best remembered for his work as a physician. His masterpiece, *Canon of Medicine*,[28] was used as a standard medical textbook for nearly six centuries in the Persian Empire and Europe. The *Canon of Medicine* comprises five large books, the first of which is about principles of physiology, anatomy, history, examination, and hygiene. In it Ibn Sina describes ear anatomy, including an explanation of the external auditory canal that protects the ear from heat and cold,

---

25 Hawkins (2004).

26 Hawkins (2004).

27 Hamidi, S., Sajjadi, H., Boroujerdi, A., Golshahi, B., & Djalilian, H. R. (2008). Avicenna's Treatise on Otology in Medieval Persia. *Otology & Neurotology*. 29(8), 1198–1203. doi: 10.1097/MAO.0b013e318187e1af.

28 Gruner, O. C. A Treatise on the Canon of Medicine of Avicenna, Incorporating a Translation of the First Book. AMS Press (1973).

Alev Uneri

and hypothesizes that sound is produced by sound waves striking nerves. According to Hamidi et al., "He seems to indicate the middle ear when mentioning a 'cavity that contains stagnant air.'"[29] Ibn Sina also describes a type of hearing loss resulting from this cavity being filled. Overall, his descriptions suggest that he had an understanding of the presence of the middle ear cavity and the shape of the cochlea.[30]

France, Shropshire, and Darwins

As you will soon realize, time moves slowly in the medical world. While the ear (outer and inner) was—and still is—recognized as the organ of hearing, it took seventeen centuries after Galen named the inner ear for the science community to discover that its membranous sacs and canals play a different role than facilitating hearing.

In the 18th century, Julien Offray de la Mettrie[31] (1709–1751), a French physician and monistic philosopher who was probably utterly unaware of the existence or function of the vestibular system and had absolutely no clue about vestibular physiology, wrote *Traité* du *Vertige* (Treatment of Verigo) (1737). La Mettrie was a military doctor who ran French field hospitals in Flanders. He was a materialist and follower of monistic philosophy, the metaphysical and theological view that all is one without fundamental divisions and that a united law lies behind all of nature. Although this philosophy looks pretty similar to the underlying principles of holistic medicine, we can't be sure he thought the same, because he didn't say (write) anything about it. His study of vertigo was purely symptomatic-based— very similar to many of today's trends in vertigo classification—and it's fair to say that its major contribution was to the history of medicine as

---

29 Hamidi, S., Sajjadi, H., Boroujerdi, A., Golshahi, B., & Djalilian, H. R. (2008). Avicenna's Treatise on Otology in Medieval Persia. *Otology & Neurotology*. 29(8), 1198–1203. doi: 10.1097/MAO.0b013e318187e1af.

30 Hamidi (2008)

31 Hacking, I. (2009). La Mettrie's soul: Vertigo, fever, massacre, and the Natural History. Canadian Bulletin of Medical History, 26(1), 179-202. DOI: 10.3138/cbmh.26.1.179.

opposed to scientific understanding of vertigo. La Mettrie published *Traité du Vertige* with a notice in the introductory pages that mentions a "Latin Dissertation in the form of a Letter," so it looks like this was his thesis for a medical degree.

In 1796, a practicing physician in Shropshire, England, wrote a book with a section on vertigo. The book was titled ZOONOMIA; or, The Laws of Organic Life,[32] and the author was Erasmus Darwin, M.D. F.R.S., also known as the grandfather of Charles Darwin. This was not his first book, and his previous one apparently had some success, as he is credited on the cover as "The author of The Botanic Garden." The book had forty sections, and the twentieth section was dedicated to vertigo. (In case you're interested, the twenty-first was about drunkenness. Perhaps he thought that they might be connected, or maybe they just had similar clinical symptoms?)

Darwin wrote a perfect description of an acute vestibular episode with auditory symptoms (possibly humming): "Violent vertigo, from whatever cause it happens, is generally attended with undulating noise in the head, perversions of the motions of the stomach and duodenum, unusual excretion of bile and gastric juice, with much pale urine, sometimes with yellowness of the skin, and a disordered secretion of almost every gland of the body, till at length the arterial system is affected, and fever succeeds."

Elsewhere he noted, "When a person revolves with his eyes closed till he becomes vertiginous, and then stands still without opening them, he seems for a while to go forward in the same direction." He categorized vertigo into three distinct types.

1. Slight vertigo

2. Auditory vertigo

3. Another kind of vertigo

He believed that "slight vertigo" affected only elderly people and was sparked by deteriorating sight and indigestion. Indigestion? Severe vertigo

---

32 Darwin, E. (1794). Zoonomia; or the Laws of Organic Life. J. Honson.

episodes are usually accompanied by nausea and vomiting, which I assume led him to believe that a problem with the digestive system could cause vertigo. One more time, everyone: Correlation is not causation. Moving on, Darwin described "auditory vertigo" as "noise in the head . . . which is also very liable to affect people in the advance of life and is owing to their hearing less perfectly than before."

The definition of "another kind of vertigo" is as vague as its classification name. Darwin wrote that it "begins with the disordered action of some irritative muscular motions, such as those of the stomach from intoxication." I'm sure you'll agree it's not what you would call a great classification, but it is a good observation from a great thinker, and between you and me, it reminds me of some contemporary classifications. Seriously, if you examine some vertigo classifications closely, you'll soon see what I mean.

In the first half of the 19th century, scientists and researchers began to dissect the inner ear and try to understand its function. The French physiologist Jean Pierre Flourens broke new ground in 1824 when he discovered that damage to the semicircular canals of pigeons' ears affected their posture, balance, movement, and flight—but not their hearing.[33] This was a revolutionary discovery, because until that point it had always been thought that hearing and balance were associated; scientists had not yet discovered that different parts of the inner ear had different functions. Flourens continued to peck away at his research into the inner ear, and in 1830 he showed how stimulating each semicircular canal can cause nystagmus—a term coined only forty years previously—in its plane. His excitement at this discovery was apparently not shared by his peers. No one showed much interest in his work until Prosper Meniere came along thirty or so years later.[34]

---

33 Flourens, P. (2010). Recherches expérimentales sur les propriétés et les fonctions du système nerveux dans les animaux vertébrés. Kessinger Publishing. (Original work published 1824.) And Flourens, P. (1830). Expériences sur les canaux semi-circulaires de l'oreille. *Mémoires de l'Académie royale des sciences.*

34 Maranhão-Filho, P., Maranhão, E. T., & Marques de Oliveira. C. (2021). Prosper Menière: The man who located vertigo in the inner ear. *Arquivos de Neuro-Psiquiatria.* 79(03), 254-56. DOI: 10.1590/0004-282X-ANP-2020-0371.

At the same time as Flourens was conducting his experiments on pigeons, a Czech anatomist and physiologist—and apparently all-round genius— named Jan Evangelista Purkinjě[35] published the results of his experiments on vertigo. He used only himself as his subject, and it's safe to say that no ethics committee in the modern world would have issued approval for his methods. He created a rotary chair that he used to understand the effects of rotation while he sat in the chair with his head in different positions. Erasmus Darwin had written that when someone stops after rotating for a period round the body axis and inclines their head, the virtual motion of their surroundings changes from horizontal to vertical. Purkinjě established that the virtual motion of a person's surroundings is determined by the position of the head. His findings became known as Purkinjě's law of vertigo. The principles of this law are applied in training programs for modern-day pilots who learn that in the absence of free external references, head movements may result in uncontrollable vertigo.[36]

Unfortunately, Purkinjě eventually lost interest in vertigo. He had a dizzying array of research interests, and I suspect he was a polymath genius.

Purkinjě was followed by Adam Politzer (1835–1920), who is considered the most influential person in otology of his time (beginning of the 20th century).[37] His biographer, Albert Mudry, states that he is certainly one of the greatest otologists in history, and his influence on fifty years of otology research and knowledge has yet to be equaled.[38] In addition to writing his legendary otology atlas and textbooks, he invented the Politzer maneuver, which made him famous, although it is rarely used these days. He also developed a gadget called an acoumeter to assess hearing, which was used

---

35 Hawkins J. E., & Schacht J. (2005). Sketches of Otohistory part 8: The emergence of vestibular science. *Audiology and Neurotology*. 10,185–190. https://doi.org/10.1159/000085076.

36 Cavero, I., Guillon, J. M., & Holzgrefe, H. H. (2017). Reminiscing about Jan Evangelista Purkinje: A pioneer of modern experimental physiology. *Advances in Physiology Education*, 41(4), 528 –538. DOI: 10.1152/advan.00068.2017.

37 Politzer, A. (1981). *History of otology: From the earliest times to the middle of the nineteenth century*. Vol. 1. (S. Milstein., C. Portnoff, A. Coleman, Trans.) Columella Press. (Original work published in 1907.)

38 Mudry, A. (2000). The role of Adam Politzer (1835-1920) in the history of otology. *American Journal of Otology*. 21(5), 753-63. PMID: 10993470.

for more than sixty years. In 1871, Politzer became extraordinary professor at the Clinic of Otology in Vienna—the first establishment in the world to deal solely with otology—and in 1873, he became its director with Josef Gruber.[39]

Politzer was a man who acknowledged his peers and colleagues.[40] He wrote about Flourens in his *History of Otology* that "the realization that the vestibular and semicircular canal structures are not organs of sound perception, that sound perception is transmitted solely through the cochlea, is the single most important result of Flourens' experiments."[41] Still, it took more than sixty years and a man named Julius Ewald to fully understand semicircular canals' functions.

Julius R. Ewald was a German physiologist to whom we owe much of what we know about vestibular functions. He used pneumatic pressure to excite the semicircular canals of awake pigeons and recorded their eye movements—that is, he induced and measured nystagmus in them. His observations formed the foundation of knowledge about nystagmus in vestibular physiology and became known as Ewald's laws.[42]

Josef Breuer (1842–1925), a physiologist and distinguished practicing physician in Vienna, followed in the footsteps of Flourens and studied the functions of the semicircular canals in pigeons in his spare time.[43] (Breuer is possibly better known for his important role in the evolution of psychotherapy. During 1880–82, while treating a patient known as Anna O., he developed the "talking cure," which became the foundation of modern psychoanalysis. Breuer introduced Anna O. and his talking cure method

39 Young, J. R., & Mudry, A. (2020). A centennial tribute to the Politzer acoumeter. *Hearing, Balance and Communication.* 18(2), 143–148. https://doi.org/10.1080/21695717.2020.1795436.

40 Mudry (2000).

41 Politzer (1981).

42 Ewald, J. R. (1892). *Physiologische Untersuchungen Über das Endorgan de Nervus Octavus.* Bergmann JF, Publisher.

43 Hirschmüller, A. (1989). *The life and work of Josef Breuer: Physiology and psychoanalysis.* New York University Press. And Hawkins, J. E., & Schacht, J. (2005). Sketches of otohistory. Part 8: The emergence of vestibular science. *Audiology and Neurotology.* 10(4), 185-190. DOI: 10.1159/000085076.

to Sigmund Freud, and the rest is history.[44]) His first publications, in 1873–1875, were about the flow of endolymph (a clear fluid found in the inner ear's membranous labyrinth) in the semicircular canals in response to changing head movements. And later, in 1889, he suggested that otoliths on the utricle and saccule (calcium carbonate crystals on top of the inner ear cellular pads) put extra weight on the underlying hair cells and so slight shifts in them provoked by the moving of the head might be enough to allow someone to perceive the changing positions. (See Chapter 3 for more on this.)

Meanwhile, the physicist and philosopher Ernst Mach (1838–1916)[45] was conducting similar experiments on birds and fish, blissfully unaware of Breuer's work (and the pigeons near Mach were the happiest). Not only were Breuer's and Mach's papers published almost simultaneously (Breuer's in 1874, and Mach's in 1873), but they also reached similar conclusions. The two men noted that the vestibular organs are linked only to the postural equilibrium and head positions. Their findings broke new ground in the field of vestibular physiology. Personally I'm still curious about Ernst Mach's cyclostat, a device he created to observe the responses of birds and fish to angular acceleration. I can imagine birds spinning in this device— sorry, birds, it was for science!—but fish? And how could he tell that the fish's hearing was not affected?

Anyway, both Breuer and Mach were right about the vestibular organs. But afterward, "spinning" became a favorite way for the medical community to understand and explain vestibular function.

Around the same time as Mach and Breuer were drawing similar conclusions about the vestibular system, Alexander Crum Brown (1838–1922), a Scottish organic chemist, published the findings of his research on the

---

44 Pollock, G. H. (1968). The possible significance of childhood object loss in the Josef Breuer-Bertha Pappenheim (Anna O.)-Sigmund Freud relationship (I. Josef Breuer). *Journal of the American Psychoanalytic Association..* 16(4), 711-739.A

45 Hawkins & Schacht (2005).

Alev Uneri

semicircular canals.[46] He was a man of his time, and so he used a rotating table for his experiments, but unlike Mach and Breuer, he used human subjects rather than animals. After many exhausting (for both Brown and his patients) but meticulous studies, he accurately identified the physiological working mechanism of the semicircular canals.

Despite the significance of Brown's findings, I have encountered very few OHNS specialists who know his name, but almost all are familiar with Robert Bárány (1876–1936), our next pioneer.[47] Bárány, who was of Hungarian extraction but was born in Austria, was a member of Adam Politzer's famous otology clinic. In those days, external ear irrigation was the standard way to treat Meniere's disease at the clinic, and Bárány discovered that if the water was too warm or too cold, it would elicit nystagmus. He subsequently created the caloric test, which is still one of the staple tests used in diagnosing vestibular function. Bárány was awarded the Nobel Prize in physiology and medicine in 1914. At that time, he was in a prisoner of war camp in Russia, but with the help of the Nobel committee and a touch of diplomacy, he was released and received his prize in Stockholm in 1916. You may think that was a very happy and victorious period for him, but when he returned to Vienna, his critics managed to prevent his being awarded a professorship. In 1917, he moved to Sweden, where he was appointed professor of otology at Uppsala.

The discovery of streptomycin gave another boost to vestibular research.[48] In 1943, a twenty-year-old postgraduate research assistant named Albert Schatz was working in Rutgers University's soil microbiology laboratory under the direction of the renowned scientist Selman Waksman.[49] Schatz

---

46 Brown, A. C. (1874). The Sense of Rotation and the Anatomy and Physiology of the Semicircular Canals of the Internal Ear. *Journal of anatomy and physiology.* 8(Pt 2), 327–331. https://pubmed.ncbi.nlm.nih.gov/17231027.

47 Bárány, R. (1907). Physiologie und Pathologie des Bogen Gangapparatus beim Menschen. Deu Ticke.

48 Kingston, W. (2004). Streptomycin, Schatz v. Waksman, and the balance of credit for discovery. *Journal of the History of Medicine and Allied Sciences.* 59(3), 441-62. https://www.jstor.org/stable/24632177.

49 Woodruff, H.B. (2014). Selman A. Waksman, winner of the 1952 Nobel Prize for physiology or medicine. *Applied and Environmental Microbiology.* 80(1), 2-8. DOI: 10.1128/AEM.01143-13.

had isolated two different microorganisms that excreted a substance that stopped the growth of tubercle bacillus and several other penicillin-resistant bacteria. He named the substance streptomycin. There is much more to the story about the discovery of streptomycin, but it is outside the scope of this book. However, I recommend you look it up when you have a few minutes to spare.

By 1944, the United States Army was experimenting with streptomycin in military hospitals to treat life-threatening infections resulting from combat wounds. Streptomycin's effectiveness against tuberculosis had been proven by this point and it began to be used worldwide to treat infection. Soon after its widespread adoption, an extraordinary side effect emerged. Nearly 90% of the first people who received streptomycin treatment for tuberculosis became vertiginous and ataxic (they exhibited unusual, uncoordinated movements). Researchers subsequently discovered that streptomycin damaged vestibular hair cells. At the time, this caused much distress, as it was believed that sensory cells in the auditory and vestibular systems do not regenerate. However, in 1993, Taylor A. Forge[50] published the results of research that showed hair cells reappearing after aminoglycoside antibiotics (same class of antibiotics with streptomycin) had triggered their loss. Although this finding is not directly related to vertigo, it played a critical role in developing the future understanding of vestibular histology and physiology.

It should be clear to you by this stage that knowledge accumulates very slowly in the world of medicine, and new ideas and perspectives often met with some resistance. Every single advance that has been made is the result of hard work and persistence. It took us more than two millennia to move from Aristotle's resonant space idea to understanding the complex inner ear functions—and we have a long way to go. Let's hope it doesn't take two more millennia to get there.

---

50 Taylor, R. R., Filia, A., Paredes, U., Asai, Y., Holt, J.R., Lovett, M., & Forge, A. (2018). Regenerating hair cells in human vestibular sensory epithelia. eLife. 7. doi: 10.7554/eLife.34817.

CHAPTER 3

SO, WHAT IS THIS VESTIBULAR SYSTEM OF WHICH YOU SPEAK?

Action is at the bottom a swinging and flailing of the arms
to regain one's balance and keep afloat.
– Eric Hoffer

To understand vertigo/dizziness, we must learn a bit about the vestibular system. (Although you're welcome to skip this part if it doesn't pique your interest, let me tell you, it's ancient!)

The vestibular system is one of the phylogenetically oldest reflex pathways. Obviously, nobody wanted to stumble into the mud, so an advanced system was developed and gave them the freedom to swim, stroll, and fly all over the world.

Primarily, the vestibular system serves to stabilize posture and maintain balance across all vertebrate species, from fish to mammals. In more advanced vertebrates, it not only aids in orientation but also coordinates the intricate, combined movements required for navigating the air, sea, and land. The vestibular system is a marvelously complex sensorineural organization, enabling communication among the peripheral vestibular organs, visual system, proprioceptive system, brainstem, cerebellum, and cortex. Does it sound dizzyingly complex? Because it truly is!

How Hard Can It Be to Roam?

In order to fly, all one must do is simply miss the ground.
– Douglas Adams

Maybe flying is as easy as Douglas Adams stated, but moving on the earth and keeping balance is a tad more intricate.

The balance system of mammals has complex input sources to accomplish its function. These input systems are incredibly intricate, given the critical role of balance in survival and its ancient origins. Simplifying it down to the fundamental inputs, they are the visual, proprioceptive (somatosensory), and vestibular systems.

The visual system encompasses the entire visual pathway, from the eyes and ocular pathways to the oculomotor nuclei and the occipital cortex. It provides awareness of our visual surroundings, allowing us to detect changes and helping us navigate in our environment. When we move our heads, our eyes move in accordance with a reflex arc, called the vestibulo-ocular reflex (VOR). VOR acts to conduct the gaze during head movements. This reflex, activated by the vestibular system, stabilizes our gaze during head movements, ensuring that the images on our retinas remain steady and our perception of the world remains stable. For example, if the head moves to the right, the eyes move to the left, counteracting the motion, and the image stays stable even though the head has turned. (Fig. I) Since slight head movements are constant, VOR works tirelessly to stabilize the vision.

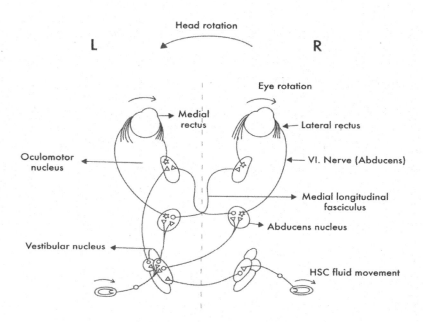

Figure I Vestibulo Ocular Reflex Arc

The second crucial component of balance perception is the propriocep-tive system, often anointed as the "sixth sense," an accurate and pretty cool name. Proprioception involves the awareness of self-movement and body position relative to the surrounding environment. Its information collec-tors are mechanosensory receptors, or proprioceptors, found in tendons, joints, and muscles. These receptors continuously transmit inputs related to muscle stretch, contraction, and elongation, as well as touch and pres-sure sensations and information about joint positions to the brain. This constant stream of inputs allows us to gain insights into the condition of our body parts relative to each other and the environment, even without visual cues or in total darkness.

For instance, thanks to proprioception, we instinctively know how high to step on stairs without looking. However, if something disrupts the pro-prioceptive system—such as in Tabes Dorsalis, a complication of syphi-lis—patients may struggle to maintain balance in the dark and can't stand upright when they close their eyes.

A bit of history: In the 1890s, Sherrington[51] coined the term "propriocep-tion" to distinguish it from exteroception and interoception. The term, derived from Latin "proprius," meaning "one's own," aptly captures the essence of feeling our bodies as our property.

Now, onto the third component of the balance function: the vestibular system. This system's end-organ is known as the labyrinth, with two laby-rinths in the skull's temporal bones mirroring each other. Each labyrinth hosts two sets of sensory receptor systems: the semicircular canals and the utriculus and sacculus pair. Three semicircular canals, oriented roughly 90 degrees to one another in all three spatial planes, are present in each labyrinth. (Fig II)

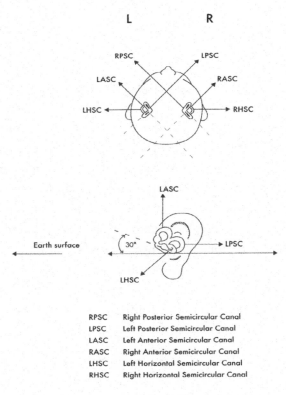

RPSC	Right Posterior Semicircular Canal
LPSC	Left Posterior Semicircular Canal
LASC	Left Anterior Semicircular Canal
RASC	Right Anterior Semicircular Canal
LHSC	Left Horizontal Semicircular Canal
RHSC	Right Horizontal Semicircular Canal

Figure II Semicircular Canals

51 Sherrington's concept of proprioception. V. Evarts, *Trends in Neurosciences*. Volume 4, 1981, pages 44-46.

What sets the vestibular system apart from the other balance-associated systems is that it doesn't rely on external cues for orientation. Instead, it evaluates motion based on the inner space of the organism. Remarkably, the vestibular system operates ceaselessly, sending data to the brain even during sleep.

Each labyrinth has afferent pathways that carry inputs to the upper centers of the central nervous system. These pathways include nuclei that serve as connection stations between them. Additionally, there are efferent pathways from the central nervous system to the lower systems, which carry outputs to the musculoskeletal system. Simultaneously, some of these pathways carry information to the cerebellum and cerebral cortex for feedback. This intricate network forms the basis for posture and gaze control, ensuring a stable background for visual perception.

All inputs from these three main sensory systems (visual, proprioception, and vestibular) are then integrated with the brainstem and cerebellum. Also, areas of the cerebral cortex, such as the occipital, parietal, and frontal cortex, play significant roles in this integration process. As a result of these arduous and complicated processes, successful motor and perceptual output arises, and we (and all other vertebrates) can merrily fly, swim, or stroll all around the world.

How Does the Vestibular System Work Anyway?

The primary function of the vestibular system is to detect the position and movement of our head in space. Each labyrinth has two sets of sensory receptor systems: semicircular canals, utricle, and saccule. These structures are filled with a fluid called endolymph, and it moves when the organism moves. Each semicircular canal, utricle, and saccule has organelles composed of sensory hair cells settled in them.

The head's rotation in various planes and angular acceleration is sensed by the six semicircular canals. These canals are arranged in three pairs, located within both temporal bones, serving as mirror images of each other. Within the temporal bone, these canals form right angles with one another. Near the opening to the utricle, each semicircular canal widens, housing a neuroepithelial structure known as the "cupula." This cupula is a gelatinous organelle containing sensory hair cells embedded within its structure. Each hair cell comprises one long "kinocilium" and 100 to 200 short "stereocilia" hairs set within the gelatinous body of the cupula. (Fig III)

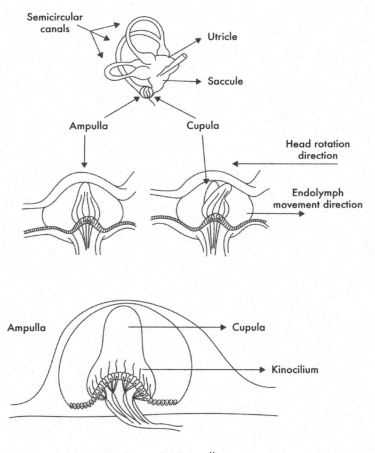

Figure III Ampulla

As the head moves, the endolymph within the semicircular canals also moves, causing the hairs (cilia) of the hair cells to bend. This bending results in a change in action potentials based on the direction of stereocilia bending. When stereocilia deviate toward the kinocilium, the resting action potential of the hair cell increases. Conversely, bending the stereocilia away from the kinocilium leads to a decrease in the action potential. It's important to note that each labyrinth is positioned as a mirror image of the other. Therefore, the same movement causes opposite-side bending of each cupula, resulting in action potentials increasing on one side and decreasing on the other. This asymmetry is interpreted as "motion" within the central nervous system.

When the motion or acceleration of the head ceases, hair cells return to their baseline positions. (Fig IV) (Fig V).

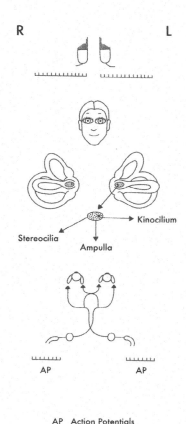

AP Action Potentials

(Fig IV) Vestibular System at Rest

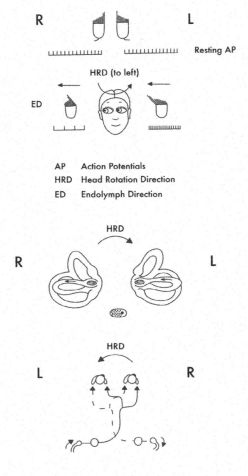

(Fig V) Vestibular System in Head Rotation

On the other hand, the utricle and saccule are responsible for sensing gravity-related motions. They sense linear accelerations and head tilting.

The sensory epithelium of the utricle and saccule have a different configuration than the cupula of the semicircular canals. Similar to the semicircular canals' cupula, there are pillow-like, gelatinous organelles in the saccule and utricle, called the macula. However, a key distinction is the presence of blankets of calcium carbonate crystals (otoliths) on each macula. These otoliths serve to detect head tilting and motion acceleration related to gravity. The utricle's macula and the saccule's macula are perpendicular to each other, enabling the utricle to perceive horizontal accelerations and the saccule to perceive vertical accelerations.(Fig VI).

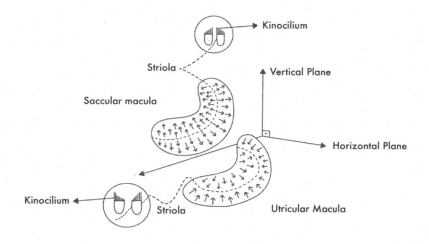

*Arrows show kinocilium orientation

Figure VI Utricular and Saccular Maculae

You may ask why the cupulas of the semicircular canals don't perceive horizontal and perpendicular motions and accelerations, and the answer is very cool: the endolymph, the cupulas, and maculae have the same density, so accelerations related to gravity don't affect them; however, the presence of otolith blankets adds weight on to the maculae, rendering them sensitive to gravity.

While no distinct anatomical boundary exists, we divide the vestibular system into peripheral and central components for clinical convenience.

The peripheral vestibular organ constitutes the outermost part, containing the semicircular canals, vestibule, saccule, and the vestibular nerve extending up to the vestibular nuclear complex. Signals from this peripheral organ reach the vestibular nuclei complex, the initial processor, and then transmit to various parts of the central vestibular system, including specific regions of the cerebral cortex, cerebellum, thalamus, and hippocampus. In these areas, afferent signals are processed, and efferent signals are adjusted to coordinate eye movements through the vestibulo-ocular reflexes (VOR) and to regulate postural control via the vestibulo-spinal reflexes (VSR).

These connections are crucial in coordinating eye movements, maintaining posture, and balancing the body. Additionally, the involvement of the hippocampus aids in spatial memory.

The central vestibular system first controls the compatibility of the data flowing from the three peripheral main systems (visual, proprioception, and vestibular) described before and picks the most available and trustworthy ones at that moment. For example, imagine you are riding on a roller coaster; the most trusted data at that moment would be the proprioceptive data coming from your sitting area, let's say, I mean from your bottom.

Creating balance would be much easier if plenty of trustful data were available. When the trustful data is insufficient, maintaining balance becomes harder. Imagine walking into an unknown room in total darkness with a thick carpet. Total darkness leaves you without visual clues, and the thick carpet makes proprioceptive data harder to trust.

Usually, it is easier to solve a balance problem with fewer data rather than ample but conflicting data. I suggest also giving an example for this condition; imagine you are in a boat on a stormy day. Your vestibular system will tell you are rocking (which is very accurate in this case), your visual system will tell you the horizon line is moving up and down (relatively true), and your proprioceptive system will tell you are standing on a very stable hard surface, which is the boat's floor (also very true), and this is a hard problem to solve for the central balance system. For many, including myself, this situation stays unsolvable, leaving them barfing and questioning themselves: what (the hell) did we think while getting on a boat?

In a resting state, all vestibular end-organs (cupulas and maculae) continuously send electrical information, known as resting action potentials, to the central nervous system. When motion occurs, this information changes.

Any head motion, except for linear acceleration, induces movement of the endolymph in at least two semicircular canals; in complex rotations, four or six canals may be affected. These interactions always occur conversely between the right and left sides. Due to the mirror symmetry of the semicircular canals, when one side bends and increases action potentials (hyperpolarization), the opposite side's bend creates a decrease (depolarization). Consequently, both vestibular nerves transmit different (asymmetric) messages to the upper centers, interpreted as a turning movement of the head (with the turning sensation towards the side with decreased impulse).

While this information may seem unnecessary or excessive at first glance, it is crucial to understand why and how dizziness occurs.

When the World Starts to Spin (Beyond Universal Studios)

In our daily lives, the vestibular system senses actual motion. In contrast, vertigo (subjective perception of virtual motion without actual movement) is simulated by the vestibular system when driven by a proper stimulus.

We looked at the basics of how the vestibular system works; now, let's explore what happens when the vestibular system malfunctions.

In a healthy vestibular system, the resting potentials of both sides are symmetrical. Based on previously stored data, any pathological condition causing asymmetry would be interpreted as a movement by the upper (central) vestibular centers. This interpretation (there is a movement) is then compared with data from the other two main balance sources: vision and proprioception. However, in that case, the corresponding checks from the other two primary data sources won't be congruent (because there is no actual movement), which leads to sensory dissonance within the vestibular system.

When the central vestibular system interprets vestibular asymmetry as motion, it immediately sends impulses to the visual and proprioceptive systems, expecting corresponding movement. However, since there is no actual movement, the eye reaction creates nystagmus (VOR), and proprioceptive discordant response causes stumbling (VSR). Since the electrical discharges from semicircular canals are more intense than the utricle and saccules' inputs, the patient usually perceives the illusion of motion as spinning. (Fig VII)

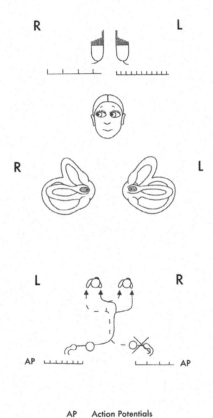

AP   Action Potentials

Figure VII Vestibular Asymmetry Due to the Hypoactivity of the Right Labyrinth

Nystagmus: The Skipping Eyes!

When we move our heads, our eyes move too by a reflex arc called the vestibulo-ocular reflexes (VOR). The vestibular system activates this reflex arc to control the gaze during head movements. The goal is to stabilize the images on the retinas, creating a stable background for us. If VOR doesn't work, our world becomes wobbly with every movement we make.

For example, when we move our head to the right, our eyes move to the left, stabilizing the image even as we turn our heads. Since small head movements are always present, VOR continuously stabilizes vision.

While this reflex helps maintain a stable world in health, things change when a vestibular problem occurs. Asymmetric discharge from vestibular end organs activates the VOR, causing the gaze to shift slowly to an imaginary new sideways position, similar to when we turn our heads. When the eyes reach their anatomical motion limits, the gaze abruptly returns to its original position, only to slowly shift again to the imaginary sideways position due to continuing asymmetric vestibular discharge resulting from the pathologic condition. However, since there is no corresponding head movement, only the eyes move spontaneously and continuously. As a result, the patient perceives the world as spinning when they open their eyes. These slow and fast eye movements are called nystagmus, with the direction of the fast movement defining the direction of the nystagmus.

The pathological asymmetric discharge of the labyrinth also activates the anterior horn cells of the spinal cord via the vestibulospinal reflex arc (VSR), attempting to correct body posture based on the expected movement (which isn't there). Again, conflicting data leads to imbalance and stumbling.

If the pathological discharge is strong enough, it may also stimulate the dorsal efferent nuclei of the 10th cranial nerve (Vagus). This activation results in hyperactivity in the intestines, leading to symptoms such as nausea, vomiting, cold sweats, and tachycardia. Thus, the entire picture of a vestibular episode is complete.

A Reeling Memory

I vividly recall an image from my childhood: my auntie, besieged by one of her debilitating migraine attacks, was seated in her favorite armchair, a bandana tightly secured around her forehead, her temples compressed in a desperate bid for relief. Tears streamed down her cheeks, and I filled with a sense of helplessness, watched on, wishing I could ease her suffering.

Years passed, and I was in medical school; one day, I returned home to discover her immobilized by a severe vertigo attack. It was my first encounter with such a phenomenon. Yet, the textbooks and classes had prepared me well—I recognized the telltale signs of positional nystagmus. I could be able to relieve her and myself that it was a benign condition, but the image was etched into my mind like a looping GIF of nystagmus.

At that point, I wasn't aware of the correlation. Still, as I began working with vertigo patients, I encountered many who, like her, experienced their first vertigo episodes after menopause had freed them from their migraine crises.[52]

That memory and experience—a connection between two seemingly disparate conditions—helped to broaden my understanding of vestibular disorders and fuel my determination to alleviate the suffering of others.

The Single Labyrinth Fallacy!

It is easy to underrate the importance of a sensory system
whose receptor is buried deep within the skull
and of whose performance we are usually not aware.
– Wilson and Melvill Jones

---

52 Lempert T, Neuhauser H, Daroff RB (2009). Vertigo as a symptom of migraine. *Ann NY Acad Sci.* 1164:242–251.

The quote above is from Wilson and Melville's book, *Mammalian Vestibular Physiology*, published in 1979. Sadly, this statement remains relevant today. Kingma and Van De Berg[53] wrote, "…as many doctors are unaware of the relevance of the vestibular system in daily life and also think that central compensation and sensory substitution almost completely deal with vestibular loss and reduce complaints to a minimum. Also, in unilateral loss, it is often affirmed that the healthy labyrinth will take over. How absurd such a statement is, becomes clear if we claim that losing one ear or one eye is of no importance as we can still hear with one ear and see with one eye. Losing one vestibular organ, like losing one ear or eye, results in a disturbing asymmetry."

More imprudently, many physicians believe that sacrificing one side of the vestibular system in the name of treating Meniere's disease is acceptable, assuming the healthy side will compensate for the sacrificed one. Surgical procedures, such as vestibular neurectomy or aminoglycoside injections into the middle ear, were invented to target "intractable" vertigo by severing the vestibular nerve or damaging the inner ear. These procedures are based on the assumption that the healthy side will compensate for the sacrificed one.

This belief stems from the misunderstanding of the vestibular system's compensation mechanisms. Many physicians assume that compensation mechanisms can fully offset vestibular loss, particularly in cases of unilateral disease. Consider the absurdity of expecting the whole vestibular system to function normally despite one side being compromised.

Just imagine one side of your vestibular system isn't functioning properly, yet you expect this highly intricate and sensitive system to continue as if nothing has changed. Consider how ludicrous it would be to claim that losing one ear or eye isn't significant, and you may not notice the difference! It's simply absurd. Professionals and those around these patients should take this matter seriously.

---

53 Kingma H., Van De Berg R., Anatomy, physiology, and physics of the peripheral vestibular system. *Handbook of Clinical Neurology*, Vol. 137 (3rd series) Neuro-Otology, Elsevier, 2016.

If you're a physician, listen attentively to your patients. And if you're a friend or a spouse, lend a compassionate ear when they speak of their suffering. Show empathy, show sympathy, and most importantly, believe them. Let's reject the notion that vestibular loss is trivial and instead acknowledge its profound impact on daily life.

Another critical fact often overlooked by professionals is the long-term trend of Meniere's decreasing vertigo episode frequency, coupled with an increased likelihood of involvement of the contralateral ear.[54] Research indicates that in at least 40% of cases, the condition progresses to bilateral disease in the long run.[55] Therefore, at least 40% of patients who undergo destructive procedures are at risk of bilateral vestibular hypofunction.

Losing function in both vestibular end-organs lacks a common term in lay language, unlike "deafness" or "blindness," despite being a substantial handicap. Bilateral vestibular function loss (bilateral vestibular areflexia) often goes unrecognized, leaving patients feeling helpless.

54 Huppert D., Strupp M., Brandt T., Long-term course of Menière's disease revisited. *Acta Oto-Laryngologica*. 2009, Volume 130, Issue 6.

55 David B., Catrin B., et al. Endotype-Phenotype Patterns in Meniere's Disease Based on Gadolinium-Enhanced MRI of the Vestibular Aqueduct, *Front Neurol*. 2019; 10: 303.

CHAPTER 4

THE NAME GAME

If somebody thinks they're a hedgehog,
presumably you just give them a mirror and a few pictures
of hedgehogs and tell them to sort it out for themselves.
– Douglas Adams

Quantum Weird Patients (Not Particles, Although That Too!)

Some diseases are typically defined and diagnosed in medicine based on their clinical symptoms. Therefore, each clinical symptom cluster related to vertigo or dizziness is designated according to its characteristics. For instance, extended dizziness is termed chronic dizziness, bursts of vertigo triggered by sudden head movements in specific positions are identified as benign paroxysmal positional vertigo (BPPV), and a severe vertigo episode following a viral infection is commonly referred to as vestibular neuritis, among other specific designations. When examining the medical literature, one encounters hundreds of thousands of papers and textbooks dedicated to vertigo, dizziness, and related topics. In the majority of these publications, various categories of vertigo are outlined. Such categorization proves immensely beneficial, fostering a shared understanding and vocabulary among professionals.

I started work at Marmara University's Neurologic Sciences Institute (MUNSI) in 1995. While the name might evoke images of a sleek "Institute" constructed with steel and glass (as it did for me), the reality was quite different. I vividly recall the vast prairie outside my window, transforming into golden chaff during the dry summer, with occasional sightings of horses passing by. It dawned on us that these horses weren't stray; they belonged to gypsies living in our neighborhood who occasionally pilfered our telephone wires (made of copper and worth stealing). Consequently, we had to rely on personal mobile phones to stay connected with the outside world.

Although the external setting of the Institute presented challenges, the internal dynamics were just the opposite. Perhaps it didn't exude the "futuristic" vibe one might expect, but it proved more than sufficient. The individuals working there were a cohort of ambitious, young, dedicated hard workers committed to the profound mission of "saving lives."

MUNSI's foundation was rooted in neurosurgery, affiliated with the MU neurosurgery department, and led by one of the world's eminent neurosurgeons, Dr. N. Pamir, who was the head of the department and the institute.

Shortly after embarking on the journey to set up a vestibular clinic in an old mice Airbnb, a remarkable colleague descended like a blessing. Let me introduce Ayfer Kucukmetin, M.Sc., a vibrant and exceptionally bright audiology specialist. She was my assistant and colleague, became my right arm and close friend, and remains so. Together, we embarked on a continuing journey that blended professionalism and camaraderie.

Fast-forward two years, and our records boast over twelve-hundred vertigo patients. The time had come to pen a documentation paper—a piece that classifies my patients and unravels our venture's intriguing statistics. Every vertigo clinic worldwide has similar documentation papers delineating clear-cut numbers of "who has what." So, here I am, navigating the labyrinth of data, ready to add our story to the global narrative.

I anticipated compiling numbers for Meniere's, BPPVs, vestibular neuronitis, and so on. We initiated the transfer of patient data and diagnoses onto Excel sheets, a task intended to conclude within a couple of weeks. However, it proved to be an elusive goal, as my patients didn't conform to the typical mold observed in diagnostic categories. Unlike others, they felt free to span across multiple categories, a situation that, albeit inappropriate (sigh!), was the reality we faced. This process turned out to be perplexing.

I felt immersed in a pool of peculiar data, resembling the strangeness observed in quantum physics. I refer to it as "quantum weird," because my patients seemed to behave like particles, freely existing in three different categories simultaneously. It was truly astonishing. Many reputable clinics had papers on patient "categorization," suggesting that their patients neatly fit into specific classifications. If you find my explanation challenging, consider this example: Brandt and Dietrich published an article in 1999 in the *Journal of Neurology*.[56] They presented data on 1370 patients. This information was neatly organized in a table (Table 1), providing a clear and straightforward overview.

---

56 M. Dieterich, T. Brandt. Episodic vertigo related to migraine (90 cases): vestibular migraine. *Journal of Neurology*, 1999, Springer.

VERTIGO SYNDROME	Number	Percentage
Benign Paroxysmal Positional Vertigo	258	18.8
Phobic Postural Vertigo	196	14.3
Central Vestibular Vertigo	185	13.5
Meniere Disease	101	7.3
Vestibular Migraine	83	6
Vestibular Neuritis	67	4.9
Psychogenic Vertigo (without postural phobic vertigo)	41	3
Bilateral Vestibulopathy	31	2.3
Vestibular Paroxysm (disabling positional vertigo)	24	1.8
Perilymph Fistula	3	0.2
Other Rare Cases (determined)	31	2.3
Vertigo of Unknown Etiology	64	4.7
Central Vestibular Syndromes without vertigo	186	13.6
Diseases Without Vertigo	100	7.3

Table 1. Frequency of various vertigo syndromes in 1370 outpatients of a dizziness unit (1989–1995)

As you can see, in Table 1, there are certain numbers of patients on each diagnostic category. For example, in our records, a patient may present with a BPPV episode and undergo an Epley maneuver, leading to complete recovery with no residual symptoms. The patient reports feeling excellent at the follow-up visit, typically two weeks later. However, the same patient might return one or two years later with an acute vestibular episode involving vertigo, nausea, humming in the ear, and possibly temporary sensorineural hearing loss in lower tones. After treatment, they would return for a follow-up four weeks later with no residual symptoms. Yet, six months

Alev Uneri

later, they might complain of continuing dizziness. This pattern could manifest in various combinations or be reversed.

In summary, I encountered every imaginable category combination, which left me stunned. Despite delving into the literature, I found that papers addressing this specific problem were exceedingly rare; they were as scarce as hen's teeth, and regrettably, I found nothing. Maybe I shouldn't say "nothing," because while looting the literature, I discovered how Charles Darwin hated barnacles! He spent nearly eight years of his life classifying barnacles to no avail; he summarized his feelings in a short sentence: "I hate a barnacle as no man ever did before, not even a Sailor in a slow-moving ship." I've always cherished my work and loved my patients; however, empathizing with Darwin's bitterness from desperation is not hard.

I believed "entangled patients" like the ones I've encountered might be more prevalent among vertigo cases than currently recognized. Awareness of VM would probably solve that problem by noticing the migraine basis is the common denominator among free-floating patients.

Classifying Complexity: Why Do We Need Medical Categorizations?

One might question the need to classify numerous intricate and interwoven clinical classifications. While providing a precise answer isn't straightforward, I can borrow a quote that explains a different concept but aligns perfectly with this context: "Hierarchies serve an important function. They enable complete strangers to know how to treat one another without wasting the time and energy needed to become personally acquainted."[57]

Vertigo patients pose considerable challenges for physicians, especially physicians who do not have enough time to thoroughly examine a vertigo patient or don't have the needed experience—a situation that is quite understandable. Effectively managing vertigo cases demands ample time

---

57 Yuval Noah Harari. *Sapiens: A Brief History of Humankind.*

per patient to listen attentively, conduct thorough examinations, and explain their condition comprehensively. Unfortunately, how many of us have the luxury of such time? Consequently, albeit regretfully, classifications become a necessary tool. You may ask how, so let's try Hariri's quotation, changing "hierarchies" with "classifications" and "complete strangers" with "physicians." "Classifications serve an important function. They enable physicians to know how to treat their vertigo patients without wasting the time and energy needed to become personally acquainted." See how perfectly fitted? Classifications serve as a "common language" in many fields, which enable us to understand each other. Otherwise, it would be impossible to talk in a meeting or write an article and to be understood.

Also, this paragraph from Harari's book resonates with the classification challenge in our field[58]: "In the bureaucracy, things must be kept apart. There is one drawer for home mortgages, another for marriage certificates, a third for tax registers, and a fourth for lawsuits. Otherwise, how can you find anything?" "Things that belong in more than one drawer, like Wagnerian music dramas (do I file them under 'music,' 'theatre,' or perhaps invent a new category altogether?), are a terrible headache. So one is forever adding, deleting and rearranging drawers."

I think that is what AAO-HNS[59] and IHS[60] (International Headache Society) are striving to achieve the same goal: creating a 'common language' with their extensive and intricate classification algorithms.

58 Yuval Noah Harari. *Sapiens: A Brief History of Humankind.*

59 Merchant, Saumil N.; Adams, Joe C.; Nadol, Joseph B. Jr. Pathophysiology of Ménière's Syndrome: Are Symptoms Caused by Endolymphatic Hydrops? *Otology & Neurotology:* January 2005, Volume 26, Issue 1, pp. 74-81.

60 Headache Classification Committee of the International Headache Society (IHS). The International Classification of Headache Disorders, 3rd edition (beta version). *Cephalalgia.* 2013;33:629–808.

Decoding Complexity: Occam's Razor

Entities should not be multiplied beyond necessity.
– William of Ockham

It is excruciating to admit, but this is our real problem in today's medicine: We have lost our holistic approach, which is essential for medicine, for some time. After many years, now I firmly believe it is impossible to understand our patients sufficiently without knowing the circumstances of their lives, past, relationships, and even their beliefs and habits. Ivanov[61] points it out as: "The human organism comprises various physiological and organ systems, each with its own structural organization and functional complexity, leading to complex, transient, fluctuating and nonlinear output dynamics. Basic physiology and clinical medicine widely employ a reductionist approach, and consider health and disease through the prism of the structural organization and dynamics of individual organ systems… However, the human organism is an integrated network, where multi-component physiological systems, each with its own regulatory mechanism, continuously interact to coordinate their functions. "

In summary, the human body's various systems work together in harmony, constantly interacting and coordinating to maintain good health. However, more than simply having intact and functioning systems is needed to preserve health.

This perspective holds true not only for vertigo patients but also for conditions like hypertension, diabetes, and more. Accurate understanding is crucial for providing efficacious help; otherwise, managing these conditions becomes challenging.

---

61 Ivanov, P. C. (2021). The New Field of Network Physiology: Building the Human Physiolome. *Frontiers in Network Physiology.* 1, 711–778. https://doi.org/10.3389/fnetp.2021.711778.

Although I acknowledge the logic behind creating categories, I am reminded of Francis Bacon's words[62]: "Truth will sooner come out from error than from confusion."

When health professionals confine themselves solely to classifications or algorithms, there is a risk of overlooking the reality of our patient's lives and actual problems. While classifications and algorithms are invaluable tools in medicine, it is essential to be aware of their limitations. Diagnosing a patient's vertigo without considering their genetic predisposition,[63] health history, lifestyle, eating habits, and stress levels may lead to misdiagnoses, especially regarding conditions such as vestibular migraine.

62 Aphorism 20, Book II.

63 Tak, Y., Tassone, F., & Hagerman, R. J. (2024). Case Series: Vestibular Migraines in Fragile X Premutation Carriers. *Journal of Clinical Medicine.* 13(2). https://doi.org/10.3390/jcm13020504.

CHAPTER 5

PHOENIX OF OTOLOGY: MENIERE'S DISEASE

Prosper Meniere: The Man Behind the Disorder

Surprisingly, Prosper Meniere, despite his extraordinary career and prolific writings encompassing both literary and medical realms, remains relatively obscure, even in France.

Allow me to share my hypothesis on this matter, rooted in a bit of historical gossip. In the tumultuous summer of 1830, a revolution erupted in Paris against Charles X, leading to three days of bloody street battles. Charles and the royal family had to flee to England, with Louis Philippe, Charles' cousin, chosen to reign over France instead of his grandson Henri V. During this upheaval, almost two-thousand wounded individuals from the street fighting were brought to L'Hotel-Dieu, where Meniere served as a member of the surgical team. It was a profound experience for the young surgeon, prompting him to record everything meticulously. This inference is supported by the fact that he published his first book, a substantial 368 pages, in the same year.

Fast forward to 1833, and Meniere received a significant appointment from the French government—to be the physician-in-residence to the beautiful and ambitious Duchesse de Berry. She, the widowed daughter-in-law of exiled Charles X, had fled to England with the royal family in 1830. The Duchesse de Berry, with her son Henri V (the grandson of exiled Charles X), declared her son the throne's legitimate heir in 1831 and ventured from England to Naples.

In a covert return to France, the Duchesse de Berry attempted a rebellion against Louis Philippe, a venture that ended in a "tragicomic" failure. After living in hiding for five months, she was eventually captured and imprisoned in the Chateau of Blaye. It was during this period that Prosper Meniere stepped into the spotlight as her physician, swiftly evolving into her "trusted confidante." I am quoting from Joseph E. Hawkins; "Meniere found himself serving not only as her 'medical adviser' but as a diplomatic mediator as well, between the temperamental prisoner and her stern military guardian, General Robert Bugeaud. With his charming personality, considerate attitude, and exemplary manners, Meniere soon became her trusted confidant…To keep Duchesse entertained, he took her for walks…explaining the local flora, rock formations, and fossils." A questionably good way to entertain the young, beautiful and ambitious Duchesse, in my opinion. " In the evenings, he chatted with her and her attendants about literature and music. At the same time, he was able to satisfy the government ministers in Paris with his regular reports about the state of her health and spirits…"[64]

Despite being a ten-year widow, the Duchesse surprisingly revealed she was a few months pregnant, attributing it to a recent marriage to a Sicilian diplomat during one of her visits to Palermo. However, the authenticity of this story remained dubious. Ultimately disgraced in the eyes of her

---

64 Prosper Ménière; Émile A Ménière. La captivité de Madame la duchesse de Berry à Blaye. 1833: journal du docteur P. Ménière. Paris: C. Lévy, 1882.

supporters, she was released from imprisonment, marking the end of Meniere's demanding and challenging task.

Upon his return to Paris in 1834, Meniere resumed his clinical duties. Despite earning the prestigious title of Chevalier of the Legion de Honor in 1835 for his remarkable efforts to prevent a cholera epidemic in southern France, academic recognition remained elusive. Even with notable clinical and literary achievements, Meniere faced resistance from institutions like the French Imperial Academy of Medicine. In 1837, he participated in a competition for a professorship, securing the top spot with his thesis, only to have another candidate appointed.

Misfortune struck again when he was denied a significant administrative position for central Paris hospitals, adding to the disappointment, especially since he had outranked the successful candidate. Despite these setbacks (perhaps, or who knows?), Meniere thrived as a social butterfly in the elite circles of Paris. His standing within the elite community was further elevated when he married Anne Pauline, the daughter of a renowned physicist.

However, gossip and storms continued to swirl around Meniere. In 1838, he found himself appointed to a position for which he lacked expertise, with two other highly qualified candidates overlooked. Despite facing an angry storm in professional circles, Meniere, with his usual diligence, managed to navigate through the challenges and maintain his position.

Meniere consistently aspired to join the French Imperial Academy of Medicine, showcasing himself as a prominent physician and a prolific writer. Unfortunately, societal internal politics thwarted his attempts, leading to rejection twice. His sole opportunity to present his work on the 8th of January was marred by the absence of many academy members, purportedly due to unfavorable weather conditions (though skepticism lingers).

At the age of 61, on January 8, 1861,[65] Meniere read a paper in the Imperial Academy of Medicine Paris.[66] The article was entitled, "On a particular type of severe hearing loss resulting from a lesion of the inner ear." He described his patients who had recurring vertigo and hearing deterioration episodes, so they had to be entitled apoplectiform cerebral congestion, but none of these patients had any sequelae other than deafness; therefore, it was impossible that the reason was the cerebral hemorrhage. At that time, everybody in that profession was sure that this disease is due to a cerebral problem called "apoplectiform cerebral congestion," and they were trying to treat it with customary bleedings and purgation. Meniere, however, took a revolutionary stance. He presented his cases, aiming to shift the understanding of the disease from a cerebral to an inner ear origin. Despite his efforts, he faced limited audience engagement and his presentation failed to impress the attending members, with even the committee deeming it unworthy of discussion.

Just a week later, on the 15th of January, Trousseau read a paper entitled "Concerning apoplectiform cerebral congestion in its relation to epilepsy," [67] and, quite unfairly (as I see it), he managed to initiate a discussion that spanned six weeks. Unfortunately, Meniere, not a member of the Academy, found himself in the audience without the privilege to speak. However, he had a specific interest, maybe even a vested interest. He published on the 26th of January in the Paris Medical Gazette a report of Trousseau's paper and the early discussions.[68] That was the first of five publications by Meniere on that particular subject in 1861.

He published three more papers in February, April, and June; he supported his claim that the disease known as "apoplectiform cerebral congestion" was indeed a disease of the inner ear, not the brain.

---

65 Meniere P; Atkinson M, trans. Gazette Medicale de Paris 1861. Meniere's original papers. Acta Otolaryngol. 1961;((suppl 162)).

66 Prosper Meniere (1799-1862) A Synopsis of His Life and Times Andrew W. Morrison, MB, ChB, FRCS, DLO. *ENT-Ear, Nose & Throat Journal.* September 1997 Volume 76, Number 9.

67 Trousseau A. De la congestion cerebrae apoplectiforme, dans ses rapports avec epilepsie. *Gaz. Med.* Paris 1861; 16:51

68 Meniere P. Academie de Medicine: congestions cérébrales apoplectiforme: M. Trousseau, discussion: MM. Bouillaud, Piorry, Tardieu, Durand-Fardel. *Gaz Med Paris.*1861;16:55-57.

On the 21st of September, he published his leading claim; basically, this was his original paper which he presented on January 8th in the Imperial Academy of Medicine Paris, with a changed title; "A report on lesions of the inner ear giving rise to symptoms of cerebral congestion of apoplectic type,"[69] and this is the paper referred to in publications for decades.

Would you like to read a piece from this original paper of P. Meniere from the translation of D. M'Kenzie in 1924[70]? Of course you do; we all love history, right? I give a literal translation of Meniere's account, preserving the original punctuation: "I have already spoken, a long time ago, of a young girl, who, having traveled by night in winter on the outside of a diligence, when she was at a catamenial period, had, in consequence of a considerable cold, complete and sudden deafness. Having been received into the service of M. Chomel, she manifested as her chief symptom continual vertigo, the slightest effort to move produced vomiting, and death followed on the fifth day. The necropsy showed that the cerebrum, cerebellum, and spinal cord were absolutely exempt from any alteration, but as the patient had become suddenly deaf after having always had perfect hearing, I removed the temporals in order to examine with care what could be the cause of this complete deafness, so rapidly supervening. The sole lesion I found was the semicircular canals filled with a red plastic material, a sort of bloody exudate, of which scarcely any traces were perceived in the vestibule and which did not exist in the cochlea. The most attentive search has enabled me to establish with all the precision desirable that the semicircular canals were the only parts of the labyrinth which showed an abnormality, and this consisted, as I have said, in the presence of plastic lymph replacing the liquid of Cotugno."

While immediate excitement didn't greet Meniere's insights among his colleagues, the tides soon turned. His groundbreaking work became widely known and referred to as "Meniere's syndrome" or "Meniere's disease." Although it would be satisfying to say that he got the "last laugh," this

---

69 Meniere P. Sur une forme de surdite grave dependant d'une lesion de l'oreille interne. *Gaz. Med. Paris.* 1861a; 16:29.

70 M'Kenzie D. Ménière's original case. *J Laryngol Otol.* 1924;39: 446–9.

remains impossible as Meniere passed away in 1862, unaware of the destiny his work would achieve.

But, dear reader, don't be sorry; Meniere, despite his challenging career with the Imperial Academy of Medicine Paris, likely lived a good and perhaps happy life.

One might wonder, especially considering Meniere's prominence, diligence, keen observations, and prolific science writing, why he couldn't secure enough votes to join the French Imperial Academy of Medicine, particularly after facing rejection twice. The intensity of his desire is apparent, raising the question of what might have hindered his acceptance. Reflecting on Meniere's challenges with the Imperial Academy of Medicine Paris and considering Barany's story (you'll read it, don't worry), one can't help but contemplate the darker aspects of human psychology and its potential detrimental effects on lives.

Despite Meniere's commendable hard work, ambition, and perseverance (and yes, I'm referring to his medical publications once again), as noted by Alan Kerr, who wrote—wittily—in 1989: "Shortly after that a tendency developed to give the name of Meniere's disease to everything that spins, something that still plagues otologists to this day."[71]

So, What Exactly Do We Know about Meniere's Disease?

If it looks like a duck and quacks like a duck,
we have to at least consider the possibility that we have a small
aquatic bird of the family anatidae on our hands.
– Douglas Adams

While this clever analogy holds true, diagnosing Meniere's disease is more complex. Just like identifying a bird as a duck, goose, swan, or even an

---

71 Kerr A.G. Aspects of vertigo. *Journal of the Royal Society of Medicine.* June 1990; 83:348-510.

archaeornithes (albeit a stretch), the certainty in diagnosing Meniere's disease is more challenging. While there may be vertigo, nausea, and aural symptoms such as aural fullness, tinnitus, or hearing loss, it's still not absolute to declare it a Meniere's disease case.

Contrary to the countless medical eponyms, as Alan Kerr aptly prophesied, the name Meniere enjoys worldwide recognition. It extends beyond the realm of medical professionals to reach vertigo patients, their relatives, and a broader audience familiar with even a bit about vertigo. Unfortunately, this prevalence of the Meniere name serves as an omen for those experiencing vertigo.

After Meniere's papers about his "vertigo cases," there were 13 years of silence on the subject until 1874, and in that year, Charcot[72] spoke on the description of vertigo, deafness, and tinnitus by Meniere and called it for the first time "Maladie de Meniere."

With the irony of fate, Charcot,[73] a leading neurologist of his time, lamented in 1881 just like Alan Kerr, mentioning Meniere's June 8, 1861[74] presentation, saying "Nevertheless, I believe that I might assert that in spite of these works a knowledge of the pathological condition in question has not yet entered as it ought into everyday practice. Although cases of Meniere's disease are not rare, far otherwise, at least in civil practice, they are nearly almost always misconstrued, connected as they are with more common disorders as, amongst others, with apoplectiform cerebral congestion or apoplectic stroke, epileptic petit mal, or again and chiefly with gastric vertigo." The persistence of the issue after 140 years is notable, albeit with a twist. Now, the prevailing assumption is that most vertigos are considered to be Meniere's disease.

---

72 Charcot. *Progrès méd.* Jan. 1874, nos. 4 and 5.

73 Charcot JM. *Lectures on the Diseases of the Nervous System.* Facsimile of London 1881 Edition, New York Academy of Medicine, Hafner Publishing Company, 1962.

74 Meniere P., Memoire sur des lesions de l'oreille interne dominant lieu a des congestion cerebrale apoplectiforme. *Gaz Med* Paris, vol. 16, pp. 597–601, 1861.

Moving forward, it is time to write about the 140-year journey of Meniere's disease; tracing many hypotheses about its origins and pathophysiology would make for a fascinating exploration. It provides an opportunity to delve into the evolution of medical understanding and perspectives surrounding this condition.

Friedrich Leopold Goltz was a physiology professor around 1870, and his main interest and working area was neuro-physiology.[75] He introduced the "hydrostatic" concept involving the semicircular canal's ability to perceive the head's position. In 1877, Gowers[76] wrote, "Although the theory of varying pressure of the endolymph originated by Goltz, rendered more precise by later writers, appears highly probable, its application to the details of the normal action of the canals is still surrounded by uncertainties which render it difficult to frame a satisfactory detailed explanation of the phenomena of this disease."

After the "endolymphatic hydrops" hypothesis was established by Goltz in 1870, the endolymphatic sac and Meniere's disease cause–effect relationship became the long-running hypothesis in Meniere's etiopathology.[77]

The legendary Prof. G. Portmann began his OHNS carrier in the early 20th century; he wrote: "From the beginning of my otological studies, in 1921, I was interested in the structure and the physiology of the internal ear in comparative anatomy." And after hard labor and 50,000 histopathologic specimens, he described endolymph's physiology and endolymphatic sac's role on its dynamics. He described endolymphatic sac drainage surgery for intractable vertigo patients in 1927.[78] After Portman, H.F. Schuknecht[79]

75 Young J Pentland, New York, Macmillan (Goltz), *Physiology*, by Edward Albert Sharpey-Schäfer, 1900.

76 W.R. Gowers. The Diagnosis and Treatment of Auditory-Nerve Vertigo. *Br Med J.* 1877 Mar 10; 1(845): 287–289.

77 Edward Woakes. Remarks on Vertigo and the Group of Symptoms Sometimes Called Menière's Disease. *Br Med J.* 1883 Apr 28; 1(1165): 801–804.

78 Professor George Portmann, MD. Bordeaux, France. Surgical Treatment of Vertigo by Opening of the Saccus Endolymphaticus. Arch. *Otolaryngol.* 6:309, 1927.

79 H. F. Schuknecht., Pathophysiology of endolymphatic hydrops. *Archives of Oto-Rhino-Laryngology.* Volume 212, pages 253–262(1976).

contributed to the hydrops theory in 1975 by his rupture and potassium intoxication theory of episodes, based on histological studies.

Despite various hypotheses, the lack of consensus on Meniere disease's etiology, clinical diagnosis, or treatment persists. The 1995 classification of the AAO-HNS[80] had a "Certain Meniere's disease" requiring histopathologic confirmation, a somewhat sarcastic notion of having to extract a patient's temporal bone for a definitive diagnosis. However, even with such extreme measures, certainty about the validity of the "endolymphatic hydrops" hypothesis remains elusive.[81] While widely accepted in the vertigo community, scientific papers indicate that temporal bones with endolymphatic hydrops may not exhibit clinical Meniere's syndrome. Conversely, some cases with severe endolymphatic hydrops lack vertigo symptoms. Rauch SD and colleagues[82] wrote in 1989, "These results challenge the dogma that endolymphatic hydrops per se generates the symptoms of Meniere's syndrome."

Therefore AAO-HNS changed its classification in 2015.[83] And since you don't need a—histopathologic—confirmation to be sure that your patient's problem is Meniere's disease, instead of a microscope (thank goodness!) now you need a notepad and a timer, because if the vertigo episode is shorter than 20 minutes or longer than 12 hours, are not considered "definite Meniere's"; they may fall under "probable Meniere's" or another category. While my tone may be cynical, the reality is that symptoms and their duration are currently pivotal in defining Meniere's disease. Interestingly, even low-frequency hearing loss in a patient cannot definitively prove Meniere's disease.

80 Merchant, Saumil N.; Adams, Joe C.; Nadol, Joseph B. Jr. Pathophysiology of Ménière's Syndrome: Are Symptoms Caused by Endolymphatic Hydrops? *Otology & Neurotology.* January 2005, Volume 26, Issue 1, pp. 74-81.

81 Alpay, H. Cengiz; Linthicum, Fred H. Jr.Endolymphatic Hydrops Without Ménière's Syndrome.†*Otology & Neurotology.* September 2007, Volume 28, Issue 6, pp. 871-872.

82 Steven D. Rauch, MD, Saumil N. Merchant, MD, Britt A. Thedinger, MD. Meniere's Syndrome and Endolymphatic Hydrops: Double-Blind Temporal Bone Study. November 1, 1989.

83 Lopez-Escamez J.A., Carey J., Won-Ho Chung, Goebel J.A., Magnusson M., MandalàM., Newman-Toker D.E., Strupp M, Suzuki M, Trabalzini F., Bisdorff A., Diagnostic criteria for Ménière's disease. *Journal of Vestibular Research.* 25 (2015)..

After this intro, maybe it's time to say new things and find new hypotheses. H. Yamane and M. Takayama[84] did that and wrote a paper about saccular otoconia as a cause of Meniere disease in 2010 I can't say that they created a huge stir, but J. Hornibrook[85] took that hypothesis seriously and presented a new hypothesis at the Prosper Ménière Society Meeting in 2016. His presentation was about the "contemporary evidence indicating that ruptures do not usually occur, and discuss the possibility that detached saccular otoconia is the main cause of Ménière's disease." Guess what, still no excitement, only six citations in 2020, but you know things don't always move fast in Meniere's whirlpool.

The current diagnostic criteria for Meniere's disease involve the guidelines provided by the American Academy of Otolaryngology-Head and Neck Surgery (AAO-HNS), as revised in 2015[86]:

Definite MD

Two or more spontaneous episodes of vertigo, each lasting 20 min to 12 h.

Audiometrically documented low- to mid-frequency sensorineural hearing loss in one ear, defining the affected ear on at least one occasion before, during, or after one of the episodes of vertigo.

Fluctuating aural symptoms (hearing, tinnitus, or fullness) in the affected ear.

Not better accounted for by another vestibular diagnosis.

Probable MD

Two or more episodes of vertigo or dizziness, each lasting 20 min to 24 h.

84 Yamane H, Takayama M, Sunami K, Sakamoto H, Imoto T. Blockage of reuniting duct in Meniere's disease. *Acta Otolaryngol* 2010;130:233–9.

85 Hornibrook J, Bird P. A new theory for Meniere's disease: detached saccu lar otoconia. *Otolaryngol Head Neck Surg.* 2016;156:350–2.

86 2015 Equilibrium Committee Amendment to the 1995 AAO-HNS Guidelines for the Definition of Ménière's Disease. Diagnostic criteria for Ménière's disease, Jose A. Lopez-Escamez, John Carey, Won-Ho Chung, Joel A. Goebel, Måns Magnusson, Marco Mandalà, David E. Newman-Toker, Michael Strupp, Mamoru Suzuki, Franco Trabalzini and Alexandre Bisdorff. *Journal of Vestibular Research.* 25 (2015).

Alev Uneri

Fluctuating aural symptoms (hearing, tinnitus, or fullness) in the affected ear.

Not better accounted for by another vestibular diagnosis.

We should mention other possible diseases that can display the clinical symptoms documented above.

Differential Diagnosis of Meniere's Disease [87]

- Autosomal dominant sensorineural hearing loss type 9 (DFNA9) caused by COCH gene.
- Autosomal dominant sensorineural hearing loss type 6/14 (DFNA6/14) caused by WSF1 gene.
- Autoimmune inner ear disease.
- Cerebrovascular disease (stroke/TIA in the vertebrobasilar system/bleeding).
- Cogan's syndrome. Some cases may have recurrences.
- Endolymphatic sac tumor.
- Meningiomas and other masses of the cerebellopontine angle.
- Neuroborreliosis.
- Otosyphilis.
- Susac syndrome.
- Third-window syndromes (perilymph fistula, canal dehiscence, enlarged vestibular aqueduct).
- Vestibular migraine.
- Vestibular paroxysmia (neurovascular compression syndrome).
- Vestibular schwannoma.
- Vogt-Koyanagi-Harada syndrome.

---

87 Lopez-Escamez J.A.,(2015)

In essence, there's still no medical test or tool to diagnose Meniere's disease beyond patient symptoms, leading to confusion even among medical professionals. While the classification may seem definitive and comprehensive, if you are a physician dealing with enough vertigo patients, you will realize the challenge of fitting them within the proposed limits.

On a side note, as the writer, I'll share seemingly unnecessary information because history teaches valuable lessons, and "Those who do not learn history are doomed to repeat it" (Santayana G.).

Brace yourself for the 1907[88] classification; it might ring a bell: "CLASS I. Primary Labyrinthine Lesion or Irritation. (a) An acute exudation or sudden haemorrhage into the labyrinth. This is the '(true) Meniere's disease' of all authors. (b) Chronic labyrinthine lesion, not due to the above causes. The causes of the cases of this class are usually obscure. This is the 'Meniere's disease' of some authors and the 'Meniere's symptoms' of others. CLASS II. Secondary Labyrinthine Source of Irritation. In this class of cases, labyrinthine disturbance is produced by extra-labyrinthine causes. They are chiefly tympanic in origin. This is the 'Meniere's symptoms' of all writers. It will be seen, therefore, that only cases of (true) Meniere's disease fall into Division (a) of Class I. Cases placed in Division (b) of Class I are those in which the symptoms develop, gradually, and as there is nerve-deafness in these cases a differential diagnosis can only be established between them and Division (a) on the single point derived from the history of the case, namely, as to whether the onset of the symptoms was sudden or otherwise. If cases of acute Meniere's symptoms occurring in the course of some general disease like leucocythaemia be placed in Division (a) Class I (and I can see no reason why they should not be), it seems to me that probably the estimate, as stated by Frankl-Hochwart, and suggested by Gottstein, is a good deal below the mark, for cases of leucocythaemia naturally fall into

---

88 T. Wilson Parry, On The Differential Diagnosis Between Méniére's Disease and Other Cases Exhibiting Méniére's Complex of Symptoms; With Remarks on the Practical Value of the Seton in Obstinate Cases of Both Conditions, Together with Case Illustrating the Excellent Results Obtained by Seton in the Latter Condition. *The British Medical Journal.* Vol. 1, No. 2419 (May 11, 1907), pp. 1107-1110.

the hands of the general physician rather than the specialist in otology, and might thus, per-chance, not come under his notice."

There does seem a modern consensus that Meniere's disease is a peripheral disorder of the audiovestibular system, which may have something to do with the homeostasis of the endolymphatic system, and any evaluation of the treatment for it is bedeviled by its natural history: a tendency to spontaneous remission, or an undue susceptibility to a placebo effect.

Jonathan Fishman wrote in 2018,[89] "Churchill's wartime comment on the Soviet Union (BBC, London, 1st October 1939), 'It is a riddle, wrapped in a mystery, inside an enigma'; but perhaps there is a key that could equally be applied to Meniere's disease; the cause of Meniere's disease still remains an enigma, despite some 157 years since Prosper Meniere's original observations in 1861."

In short, the actual cause of Meniere's disease remains unproven. A search on PubMed reveals over 9,000 papers written since the first paper, published in 1874.

How Would You Treat Meniere's Disease?

How would you like a taste of your own medicine, doctor?
– The Dark Knight (2008)

Exploring the strange and somewhat pitiful history of surgical attempts to treat Meniere's disease underscores why I am so persistent about obtaining a correct diagnosis. One might chuckle and say, "Come on, these stories are from the 19th century!" That's true, but can we be certain that someone in the 22nd century won't shake their head and say, "Look at the tragic measures they took to treat vertigo in the 21st century!" when reflecting

---

89 Fishman, Jonathan; Fisher, Edward; Hussain, Musheer. Ménière's disease: 'a riddle wrapped in a mystery inside an enigma.' Has the key been found? *The Journal of Laryngology and Otology* (Devon). Vol. 132, No. 9, (Sept. 2018): 763-763.

on how we handled "Meniere's disease" with all these invasive surgeries and procedures?

"Direct treatment of labyrinthine infections is a subject for the special aural surgeon. I would only here indicate that when there is evidence of an irritative process, blistering behind the ear sometimes affords very marked relief to the vertigo." This sentence was written in 1877 by Gowers.[90]

"Seven years ago, a case of Meniere's disease came under my own care. It was under my direct observation for a little over two years, during which time I tried, with much patience, every important drug that has been recommended to alleviate this distressing complaint, but to no purpose whatsoever. Driven to extremities, I determined to see what a seton would do. I published this case in *The Lancet*, and, in reference to it, it will be seen that while the seton was worn, together with keeping the patient at rest, away from his work, the result was remarkable." This treatment suggestion was from T. Wilson Parry, a London surgeon, published on May 11, 1907,[91] in the *British Medical Journal*.

If you're unfamiliar with a seton, prepare to be surprised. A seton is a slender strand of thread, a strip of gauze, a length of wire, or another foreign material threaded through the subcutaneous tissues or a cyst to create a sinus or fistula, which facilitates drainage. In 1903 Crockett[92] took out his patient's stapes; in 1904, Lake[93] and Milligan[94] performed labyrinthectomy without being aware of each other. In 1904, R.H. Parry[95] cut the cochleovestibular nerve for the first time in history; it may be considered the first

---

90 Gowers W.R. The Diagnosis, and Treatment of Auditory Nerve-Vertigo. *Br Med J.* 1877, Apr 21; 1(851): 477–478.

91 Wilson P.T., (1907)

92 Crockett EA. The removal of the stapes for the relief of auditory vertigo . *Ann Otol Rhinol Laryngol.* 1903;12:6772.

93 Lake R. Removal of the semicircular canals in a case of unilateral aural vertigo. *Lancet* 1904;1:1567-1568.

94 Milligan W. Meniere's disease: A clinical and experimental inquiry. *Br Med J.* 1904, vol 2, p 1228.

95 Parry RH. A case of tinnitus and vertigo treated by division of the auditory nerve. *J Laryngol Otol.* 1904; 19:402–6.

vestibular neurectomy. More interestingly, in 1912, Barany[96] opened his Meniere's patients' skulls, observed the dura mater, closed them back, and guess what happened? "Surprisingly," he reported excellent results afterward. Maybe we can count Barany's operation as the first sham operation (a very audacious one) for Meniere's disease?

In 1919, Ballance [97] injected alcohol into the middle ear and reported excellent results, too. But in 1926, "the great" Portmann[98] described "endolymphatic sac drainage"; since then, this operation has been performed on thousands of patients. In 1936, Mc Kenzie[99] achieved the first vestibular neurectomy, a procedure that, sadly, is still in use today. You might wonder if I sound critical of surgery—yes, I am. Since we still don't know the exact cause and mechanism of the disease, dating back to the first surgical interventions in 1877, all surgeons reported excellent outcomes after their "surgeries." Even if it's true that procedures like blistering the skin behind the auricle or implanting a seton seem to help patients "heal," there's something peculiar going on there. Of course, I'm not the only skeptic; there are many more "Don Quixotes"[100] out there.

One of these "Don Quixotes" was Nicholas Torok[101]; he reviewed 834 articles on Meniere's disease published between 1951 and 1975 and found that almost all supporters of either medical or surgical treatments declared success in 60% to 80% of patients. While there are so many various therapies that are claimed to be successful, it would seem reasonable to be a skeptic and look for the influence of some factor common to all. Torok believed that the "placebo effect" might be that common factor.

96 Bárány R. Vestibular Apparatus and Central Nervous System. *Laryngoscope*. 22:81,1912.

97 Ballance, C.A. *Essays on the Surgery of the Temporal Bone*. New York, The Macmillan Company, 1919, vol. 2.

98 Portmann, G. Le traitment chirurgical des vertiges par l'ouverture du sac endolymphatique. *Presse méd*. 34:1635, 1926.

99 McKenzie KG. Intracranial Division of the Vestibular Portion of the Auditory Nerve for Ménière's Disease. *Can Med Assoc J*. 1936, Apr;34(4):369–381.

100 Furstenberg AC. A chronicle of 100 years of otolaryngology. *Bull N Y Acad Med*. 1949 Dec; 25 (12):775-91.

101 Torok, N. Old and new in Ménière disease. *Laryngoscope*. 1977;87(11):1870-1877.

In 1981, Thomsen J., Bretlau P., Tos M., and Johnsen N.J. prepared a double-blind, placebo-controlled study.[102] They were saying, "We have demonstrated previously that the placebo effect does indeed play a significant role in the success rate of treatment of Meniere's disease and that, indeed, patients with Meniere's disease are extremely good placebo responders."

With their original words; "To investigate the placebo effect in surgery for Meniere's disease, a double blind controlled study was undertaken, comparing effects of a regular endolymphatic shunt with those of regular mastoidectomy. Thirty patients with typical Meniere's disease, selected because of unsuccessful medical treatment, participated. Patients completed daily dizziness questionnaires three months before and 12 months after surgery, with the registration of nausea, vomiting, vertigo, tinnitus, hearing impairment, and pressure in the ears. Patients were operated on at two universities, and the patients operated on at one underwent a controlled study each month at the other. At the termination of the trial, both investigators and patients gave their opinions of the efficacy of the operations. Minor differences were seen between active and placebo groups, *but the greatest difference in symptoms was found when preoperative and postoperative scores were compared: both groups improved significantly.*"

If I simplify it for non-medical readers: they conducted two different operations. In half of their patients, they performed a simple mastoidectomy, which involves opening the mastoid bone, drilling some air cells, and then closing the wound. The other half underwent the regular endolymphatic sac shunt operation. One would expect that if the endolymphatic hydrops theory is correct, patients with the endolymphatic sac shunt operation should show improvement after the procedure, while those with simple mastoidectomy should remain the same as before surgery. However, surprisingly, both groups showed significant improvement.

Mirko Tos and colleagues didn't stop there. Nine years later, they published a follow-up on these patients, and the results were impressive. They reported, "Success has been maintained in about 70% of the patients in

---

102 Thomsen J., Bretlau P., Tos M., and Johnsen N.J. *Arch Otolaryngol.* 1981;107:271-277.

Alev Uneri

both groups, with no significant differences between the two groups." This success included nearly complete alleviation of symptoms. When comparing their results with all endolymphatic sac drainage procedures in the literature, they inferred, "These rather uniform results suggest that the effect of the surgery is not specifically related to the shunt procedure per se—the effect on the inner ear, however, is probably nonspecific." In the end, they weren't condemning the surgery but highlighting the strong placebo effect, especially in these troubled patients. They warned against deluding ourselves into believing that the effect is solely the result of a specific procedure alone.[103]

Vertigo and dizziness pose considerable challenges, profoundly affecting those afflicted in their physical and psychological health. Enduring these symptoms over time may lead individuals to contemplate drastic procedures, hopeful for relief. Whether opting for interventions like vestibular nerve section or labyrinth destruction or—allegedly—less invasive methods like steroid or aminoglycoside injections into the middle ear, the efficacy of such measures remains unclear. Additionally, given the ongoing uncertainty surrounding the condition's root cause, I dissent from advocates of both destructive and non-destructive surgical strategies.

Another opposition for destructive surgery lies in the natural progress of the disease. As we know, at least 40% of cases progress to bilateral disease over time.[104] In that case, the destruction of the labyrinth (or cut vestibular nerve) on one side and the development of the disease in the previously healthy side could leave the patient with severe disability.

Thomas Brandt[105] and colleagues wrote, "In the beginning, patients become symptomatic when they develop recurrent vertigo episodes and/or fluctuating unilateral cochlear symptoms such as hearing impairment, tinni-

103 Bretlau, Paul M.D.; Thomesen, Jens M.D.; Tos, Mirko M.D.; Johnsen, Niels Jon M.D. Placebo Effect in Surgery for Meniere's Disease: Nine-Year Follow-Up. *The American Journal of Otology.* July 1989, Volume 10 (4), p 259–261.

104 David B., Catrin B., et all. Endotype-Phenotype Patterns in Meniere's Disease Based on Gadolinium-Enhanced MRI of the Vestibular Aqueduct, *Front Neurol.* 2019; 10: 303.

105 Huppert Doreen, Strupp Michael, Brandt Thomas. Long-term course of Menière's disease revisited *Acta Oto-Laryngologica,* 2009, Volume 130, Issue 6.

tus, and aural fullness. According to the clinical experience of those who manage dizzy patients, the frequency of vertigo episodes decreases over the long term, while the probability of involvement of the contralateral ear increases. Most of the available clinical studies deal with only a few or just single aspects of the syndrome. The prognosis of Meniere's syndrome and the emergence of concomitant symptoms are highly relevant for both the patients and their physicians. Valid data on the development of symptoms will help the physician to select appropriate diagnostic and treatment procedures. Furthermore, he/she will be able to more readily deal with the patient's most relevant questions about the spontaneous course of their condition." And they added something more important; "As expected, the data on the long-term course of Meniere's disease varied considerably. However, the overall large number of patients included in the reviewed studies (n = 7852) allowed us to assess the most probable long-term prognosis of the disease activity. Both the frequency of vertigo episodes and the continuous worsening of the audio vestibular function spontaneously subside within the first 5–10 years, whereas the involvement of the contralateral ear becomes more frequent the longer the disease lasts. Drop episodes are infrequent complications that spontaneously remit in most cases. There have been no large, prospective, long-term multicenter studies on the spontaneous course and the differential effects of various medical treatments as regards the prevention of Meniere's episodes or its outcome with respect to audio vestibular function."[106]

I included a section about the treatment of Meniere's disease because I believe that understanding the futile attempts to treat this disease for 150 years should prompt us to reconsider our approach. As you can observe, once Meniere's disease gained recognition within the medical community, the idea of surgical intervention emerged. Procedures like creating blisters behind the ear or placing a seton under the skin, followed by the waiting period and reporting success as "remarkably successful" might elicit a contemptuous smirk. However, it's worth contemplating that someone in the future might smirk at our current practices 150 years from now. In 1977,

---

106 David B., (2019)

Alev Uneri

Nicholas Torok published a review article based on the array of articles in world literature between 1952 and 1977 about Meniere's etiology, pathology, histology, clinical diagnosis, and treatment.[107] He wrote, "This review is concerned primarily with the treatment aspect of the literature. All the published ideas, regimens, and techniques have one significant feature in common. They all claim success but not in 100% of the cases. Recovery varies from about 60% to 80%. Those cases considered "improved" are 20% to 30%, and the rate of failure is between 10% and 25%. The diagnostic tools and capabilities have improved considerably. For treatment, except for reasonable medical or surgical palliation, nothing more can be offered than was offered a half-century ago." Nearly five-decade later, we are in the exact same situation.

To Treat or Not to Treat? That is the Question...

In Meniere's disease, no matter what drug is given,
it will eventually work if given sufficient time.
– Alan Kerr

I am going to introduce one more fascinating and highly significant research study and researcher. If you adhere to the "Primum Non-Nocere" principle, meaning "First, Do No Harm," as a physician, you will appreciate why this research holds undeniable importance for patients who are assumed to have Meniere's disease.

In 1998, Kerr A.G. and Toner J.G. published a captivating paper about patients experiencing incapacitating vertigo due to Meniere's disease, referred to them for an operation.[108] In the introduction, the authors noted that over the years, they observed an intriguing phenomenon: the patients

---

107 Nicholas Torok. Old and New in Meniere Disease. *Laryngoscope.* Volume 87, Issue11, November 1977, pages 1870-1877.

108 Kerr A.G., Toner J. A new approach to surgery for Meniere's disease: talking about surgery. Clin. Otolaryngol. 1998, 23: 263-64.

became completely free from vertigo while waiting the operation.[109] Despite the patient's willingness to proceed with the operation, the authors decided to initiate a clinical trial, deeming this a very "frequent" occurrence.

They began the trial in 1994, openly explaining surgical options and assuring patients that their vertigo wouldn't last indefinitely. Patients were given a second appointment 6 to 8 weeks later.[110] In this trial, 50% of their patients experienced dramatic improvement, and 60% avoided surgery. Kerr wrote, "This leads us to ask the question: 'Is there any place at all for the so-called conservative surgical procedures in Meniere? This trial needs to continue for a much longer period with additional cases, but maybe one should just talk about surgery, and for those who fail to settle, proceed straight to a destructive procedure. Despite all the talk about evidence-based medicine, there is still no clear evidence that sac surgery or indeed any other so-called conservative procedure has any specific effect on the progress of Meniere's disease. There is not one reported controlled trial confirming the benefits of these procedures. In addition, if one would expect 70% success from a conservative procedure and can get 60% from 'planning surgery,' there must be grave doubt about the likely surgical success rate in the remaining 10% from any of the common conservative surgical procedures. The authors suspect that one would be operating on many cases for few additional successes. There is one major problem about having this hypothesis accepted; most of those who are interested in Meniere's disease want to operate. Those who get tertiary referrals will need a lot of convincing before they risk losing their referral base by not operating on most referred cases. This is often admitted privately and even occasionally in public. But, as all surgery puts the hearing of patients at some risk, maybe cherished beliefs should be put at risk instead."

Alan Kerr continued, "Notwithstanding the vivid symptomatic picture which Meniere gave in the year 1881, there has been an indescribable confusion ever since between cases of true Meniere's disease and those

---

109 McKee GJ, Kerr AG, Toner JG, Smyth GD. Surgical control of vertigo in Ménière's disease. *Clin Otolaryngol Allied Sci.* 1991 Apr;16(2):216-27.

110 Kerr AG. *J R Aspects of vertigo.* Soc Med. 1990 Jun;83(6):348-51.

exhibiting 'Meniere's symptoms' arising from other causes; consequently, the literature of the subject is exceedingly involved and obscure."

Ironically, this "indescribable confusion" surrounding Meniere's disease persisted from the beginning; "No better means can be taken to illustrate this confusion than by giving statistics from one of our best ear hospitals in London. Dr. Wyatt Wingrave most kindly searched the records of the Central London Throat and Ear Hospital for me; the result is given in the table on page 1108." In a letter accompanying this list, Dr. Wingrave wrote, "I send you figures of Meniere's cases since 1884, the earliest register I can find. Unfortunately, but little discrimination has been made in diagnosis. The nomenclature, as you see, varies considerably, for example; Meniere's disease, a labyrinthine disease with vertigo, a labyrinthine disease with vertigo and tinnitus, labyrinthine inflammation, labyrinthine anemia, and aural vertigo. Such is the awful confusion, and only to make matters worse, the actual numbers are preposterous. The last ten years are more reliable and represent an approach to the truth. The earlier records, I feel sure, are worthless as a guide. You will notice that in three of the years, no cases were recorded. We are now much more careful in diagnosis. Many of the cases recorded are doubtless middle ear in origin and not purely labyrinthine. I have not seen or heard of a genuine pure labyrinthine case for two years." Dr. Wilson Parry wrote this comment in his report on "Excellent Results Obtained by Seton" in 1907.[111]

In the realm of Meniere" disease, the ongoing challenge persists. Without a clear understanding of its cause and mechanism, physicians rely on the age-old Hippocratic approach to diagnose patients based on their symptoms. This reality may seem surprising to those outside the medical field, but in 21st-century medicine, it reflects the stark truth. Consequently, a significant controversy surrounds diagnosing and treating patients grappling with this enigmatic condition.[112]

---

111 Wilson P.T., (1907)

112 Ruckenstein MJ. Pathophysiology of Meniere's disease. In: Ruckenstein MJ, ed. Meniere's Disease—Evidence and Outcomes. San Diego, CA: Plural Pub, 2010: Radtke A, Lempert T, Gresty MA, et al. Migraine and Meniere's disease: Is there a link? *Neurology*, 2002; 59: 1700-4.

Starting in 1877, dietary restrictions became the primary and safe choice for the initial care of Meniere's disease patients, as advocated by numerous otolaryngologists: "The influence of salicylate of soda upon the equilibrium, which I have described, suggested its use in this disease. The patient with gastric ulcer, whose case has been narrated above, thought that she was better while taking the salicylate than when taking any other medicine. Its effect, unfortunately, seems after a time to become less."[113]

These restrictions contain salt, alcohol, and caffeine intake. If you check new research, you may see an interesting list of possible trigger foods to be eliminated; for example; canned foods (because of salt and MSG), processed foods (cold cuts, deli meats), anchovies, olives, pickles, kimchi and sauerkraut, soy and Worcestershire sauces, aged cheeses, chips or crackers. There is also a suggestion of gluten restriction for Meniere's disease.[114],[115]

Because this list is essentially a one-on-one match with a migraine diet, including gluten restriction, as you will read later.

Meniere's Disease, Water, Salt, and a Little Bit of Insight

One-hundred-and-sixty-three years after Meniere's original paper, we are still clueless in finding a comprehensive etiology and a scientifically approved treatment to achieve symptomatic improvement and slow the progression of this syndrome.

Issues related to water and salt balance have been considered important in various diseases such as epilepsy, migraine, and hypertension throughout ancient and recent medical history. The same holds true for Meniere's disease, where a low-salt diet is widely used as a primary treatment option.

---

113 Gowers W.R. The Diagnosis and Treatment of Auditory Vertigo. *The British Medical Journal*. April 21, 1877.

114 Ménière disease and gluten sensitivity: Di Berardino, Federica, MD; Filipponi, Eliana, Aud, Tech; Alpini, Dario, MD; O'Bryan, Tom, DC, CCN, DACBN; Soi, Daniela, MD; Cesarani, Antonio, MD. Recovery after a gluten-free diet. *Am J Otolaryngol*. 2013, Volume 34, Issue 4.

115 Di Berardino, F; Zanetti, D; Ciusani, E; Caccia, C; Leoni, V; De Grazia, U; Filipponi, E; Elli, L. Intestinal permeability and Ménière's disease. *Am J Otolaryngol*. 03/2018, Volume 39, Issue 2.

While it is believed that low salt intake helps lower endolymphatic pressure, it is not proven, much like the endolymphatic hydrops hypothesis. However, despite the lack of a precise mechanism, dietary sodium restriction has shown benefits and has been documented by many researchers.[116]

The foundation of the low-salt regimen in Meniere's disease is rather peculiar; in the 1930s, at the University of Michigan, Furstenberg, Lashmet, and Lothrop carried out a study and presented it before the American Otological Society in 1934.[117] This study was an expanded version of Dederding's previous research.[118] They concluded that the tissues involved in Meniere's disease either have an increased avidity for sodium ions or an unusual sensitivity. Based on this, they established a treatment to reduce sodium intake and eliminate body sodium through the kidney using a diuretic.[119] The treatment achieved significant success, leading to widespread recognition and approval of a low-sodium diet and diuretic among practitioners since then.[120]

Naganuma[121] wrote in 2006: "The symptoms can be temporarily reduced by conventional treatments such as dietary and diuretic therapy, but improvement is usually followed by recurrence at different intervals. The exact mechanisms of both its occurrence and fundamental pathogenesis still remain unclear" in 2006.

116 Boles, Roger; Rice, Dale H; Hybels, Roger. Conservative Management of Ménière's Disease: Furstenberg Regimen Revisited. *Ann Otol Rhinol Laryngol.* 07/1975, Volume 84, Issue 4.

117 Furstenberg AC, Lashmet FH, Lathrop F: Meniere's symptom complex: medical treatment. *Ann Otol Rhinol Laryngol.* 43: 1035-1046, 1934.

118 Dederding D: Our Meniere treatment (principles and results). *Acta Otolaryngol (Stockh).* 16:404-415, 1931.

119 Furstenberg AC, Richardson G, Lathrop F: Meniere's disease; addenda to medical therapy. *Arch Otolaryngol.* 34:1083-1092, 1941.

120 Minor LB, et al. Meniere's disease. *Curr Opin Neurol.* 2004;17(1):9–16..

121 Naganuma, Hideaki; Kawahara, Katsumasa; Tokumasu, Koji ; Okamoto, Makito. Water May Cure Patients with Meniere Disease *Laryngoscope.* 08/2006, Volume 116, Issue 8.

In short, deliberate modulation of water intake may be the simplest and most cost-effective medical treatment for patients with Meniere's.[122-123]

As mentioned earlier, issues related to water and salt balance are also significant in migraine. Oliver Sacks highlighted this connection, and he wrote, "A number of migraine patients complain of increased weight, or tightness of clothes, rings, belts, shoes, etc. in association with their episodes." He refers from Wolff, "Some weight-gain preceded the headache stage in more than a third of the patients he (Wolff) studied; since, however, the headache could not be influenced either by experimental diuresis or hydration." [124-125]

However, the subject's historical figure is Aretaeus, who suggested fluid excretion/elimination through food for migrainous patients centuries ago. More information about his diet will be explored in the upcoming chapter on food and vertigo.

122 Shim, Timothy; Strum, David Poran; Mudry, Albert; Monfared, Ashkan. Hold the Salt: History of Salt Restriction as a First-line Therapy for Menière's Disease. *Otol Neurotol.* 07/2020, Volume 41, Issue 6.

123 P. De Luca, C. Cassandro, M. Ralli, F.M. Gioacchini, R. Turchetta, M.P. Orlando, I. Iaccarino, M. Cavaliere, E. Cassandro, and A. Scarpa. Dietary Restriction for the Treatment of Meniere's Disease. *Transl Med UniSa.* 2020; May; 22: 5–9.

124 Oliver Sacks, Migraine.

125 Schottstaedt W.W., Wolff H.G. AMA Variations in Fluid and Electrolyte Excretion in Association with Vascular Headache of Migraine Type. *Arch NeurPsych.* 1955;73(2):158-164.

CHAPTER 6

HOLD ON TIGHT!
YOUR CRYSTALS ARE
ON THE MOVE!

When discussing vertigo, benign paroxysmal positional vertigo (BPPV) typically ranks as the first- or second-most common diagnosis, alongside vestibular migraine (VM) and Meniere's disease, depending on the institution or source. BPPV is often explained in lay terms as the inner ear crystal spilling. What really is happening is that otoconia (tiny calcium crystals on top of the macula; see Chapter 3) are detaching from their regular spot on the utricle and floating around in the inner ear fluid.[126-127] In scientific terms, it's actually explained in the same way. Make of that what you will.

---

126 Hornibrook, J. (2011). Benign paroxysmal positional vertigo (BPPV): History, pathophysiology, office treatment and future directions. *Int J Otolaryngol*. 2011, Article 835671. doi: 10.1155/2011/835671.

127 Bhattacharyya, N., Baugh, R. F., Orvidas, L., Barrs, D., Bronston, L. J., Cass, S., Chalian, A. A., Desmond, A. L., Earll, J. M., Fife, T. D., Fuller, D. C., Judge, J. O., Mann, N. R., Rosenfeld, R. M., Schuring, L. T., Steiner, R. W. P., Whitney, S. L., & Haidari, J. (2008). Clinical practice guideline: Benign paroxysmal positional vertigo. *Otolaryngol—Head Neck Surg*, 139(5) pp. S47–S81. DOI: 10.1016/j.otohns.2008.08.022.

The main symptom of BPPV is sudden, sharp vertigo induced by a change in the head's position. Lying down is the most likely trigger, but it can also happen if you look up or move in other ways. BPPV can last for days, weeks, or even months. While many people recover spontaneously—that is, without treatment—from a short episode of BPPV, it can be more difficult to recover from longer episodes. Furthermore, BPPV recurs. The gaps between episodes can vary, but you can be sure that if you've experienced it once, most likely you'll experience it again at some point. Let's take a short look at how the world of science has viewed BPPV in the past century.

The Crystalizing Story of BPPV

The first descriptions of BPPV in medical literature are accredited to D. Adler[128] and Robert Bárány, but it was Bárány who first pointed out the otolith organs. Furthermore, Bárány elicited vertigo in a 27-year-old woman by turning her head from side to side in a supine position and then noted the nystagmus he saw.[129]

In 1952, the researchers Margaret Dix and Charles Hallpike presented not only a complete symptomatology of BPPV but also a provocative positional diagnostic test. They described their test as "positional nystagmus of the benign positional type."[130] You might know it better as the Dix-Hallpike maneuver. The maneuver became a staple technique for examining almost all peripheral vertigo patients.

The renowned otologic surgeon Harold Schuknecht suggested in 1962 that BPPV "might be caused by detached utricular otoconia, acting upon the

---

128 Hornibrook J. (2011). Benign Paroxysmal Positional Vertigo (BPPV): History, Pathophysiology, Office Treatment and Future Directions. *Int J Otolaryngol*. 2011, 835671.

129 Barany E. (2009). Diagnose von krankheitserch-eingungen im mereiche de otolithenapparates. *Acta Otolaryngol*. 1921;2:434–437. https://doi.org/10.3109/00016482009123103. And Hornibrook (2011).

130 Dix, M. R., & Hallpike, C. S. (1952). The pathology symptomatology and diagnosis of certain common disorders of the vestibular system. *Proceedings of the Royal Society of Medicine*. 45(6), 341–354.

cupula of the posterior semicircular canal."[131] There were no human pathological studies at that time to either confirm or challenge his declaration.
So, in 1969, he tested (that is, supported) his hypothesis by reporting baso-
philic staining (a histology term that means microscopic particles, otherwise clear and invisible under the microscope, become visible through
deep blue staining) bodies attached to the posterior semicircular canal's
sensory organ (cupula) (see Chapter 3) in deceased patients who had had
BPPV symptoms.[132] The short version is that he saw microscopic particles,
which were otoliths (inner ear crystals) stuck on the sensory organ (cupula)
of the posterior semicircular canal. You'll remember from Chapter 3 that
cupulas are placed in the semicircular canals of the inner ears and sense
the head's positional changes via their cilia. Their cilia float in the semicircular fluid. The particles Schuknecht saw on top of that organelle were
an anomaly. These were otoconial crystals that fell off their original beds
and stuck on the cupula, causing them to bend because of weight (remember, a normal cupula isn't sensitive to gravity), which results in changes in
its action potentials, thus an asymmetry between two vestibular systems
signaling, which is perceived as "movement" in the upper vestibular system, hence abnormal perception (that is, a virtual head-turning motion),
of positional vertigo.

Schuknecht named the pathology "cupulolithiasis," or cupula stones,
essentially referring to otoliths as stones stuck on the posterior semicircular canal cupula. This finding was a huge step forward in understanding
why patients became vertiginous as a result of some head positions but
not others.

Cupulolithiasis remained the dominant theory for nearly thirty years,
although it has some shortcomings theoretically, as it does not explain the
long latent period and fatigability of nystagmus (that is, the time between

131 H. F. Schuknecht (1962). Positional vertigo. Clinical and experimental observations. *Transactions of the American Academy of Ophthalmology and Otolaryngol*. Vol. 66, pp. 319–331, 1962. PMID: 13909445.

132 H.F. Schuknecht (1969). Cupulolithiasis. *Archives of Otolaryngology-Head & Neck Surgery*, vol. 70, pp. 765–778, 1969. https://doi.org/10.1001/archotol.1969.00770030767020.

the nystagmus being provoked and its actual appearance and the fact that it becomes less intense over time). Beyond theoretical shortcomings, lack of understanding of the pathophysiology delayed the resolution too.

The main weakness of Schuknecht's hypothesis, though, is that if the otoliths actually do cling onto cupulas permanently (cupulolithiasis), we shouldn't see either a delay between the provocation and display, and the fading of the positional nystagmus, both of which are characteristics of BPPV. (When you repeat a Dix-Hallpike maneuver on the same side of the body, the positional nystagmus disappears. In the medical world, we say that it exhibits fatigue.) This interesting and intriguing finding puzzled the experts for nearly ten years. If there were crystals stuck on the inner ear's sensory cells, you would expect to see the same nystagmus every time you do the same head position, but that is not the case, and after two or three repeats, the positional nystagmus disappears.

The Curious Case of Free-Floating Crystals!

While cupulolithiasis was still the pathology of choice for most health practitioners, other researchers were hard at work in search of other possible explanations. First Hall et al.[133] in 1979, and later John Epley[134] in the 1980s, proposed a hypothesis of free-floating particles in the posterior canal, which Epley called canalolithiasis. In his model, otoliths floated in the semicircular canals instead of clinging to cupulas.

The otoconia are separated from the macula and spilled in the fluid-filled inner ear spaces. In their normal turnover process, these spilled otoconia are absorbed and cleaned in the macula. However, sometimes massive otoconia spills happen. If these spilled otoconia make it as far as the semicircular canals, they usually accumulate in the posterior semicircular canal

133 S. F. Hall, R. R. Ruby, J. A. McClure. (1979) The mechanics of benign positional vertigo. *Journal of Otolaryngology*, vol. 8, pp. 151–158, 1979. PMID: 430582.

134 Epley J (1979) New dimensions of benign paroxysmal positional vertigo. *Otolaryngology–Head and Neck Surgery*. 88 (5); 599–605. https://doi.org/10.1177/019459988008800514.

(PSC) because, anatomically, the PSC's ampulla (cupula's nest) is at the lowest part of the inner ear. Studies show that in 88% of BPPV cases, the affected canal is PSC, and only in 13.6% of cases are the horizontal semi-circular canals (HSC) affected.[135] The superior semicircular canals (SSCC) can also be affected, although this is much less likely.[136]

This model perfectly explained the latency and fatigue problems associated with the Dix-Hallpike maneuver. It's a little bit like playing with a snow globe. It takes time for the particles to gather at the bottom of a snow globe (just as it takes time for the particles in the semicircular fluid to move to their new venue)—that explains the latency. And if you rotate a snow globe repeatedly, fewer and fewer particles flow (most of the particles cling to the floor and stop floating at some point)—that explains the fatigue (or fading) of the positional nystagmus and vertigo when you keep repeating the Dix-Hallpike maneuver.

Like Prosper Meniere, John Epley was a bit of an underdog in the OHNS community, not least because he had dared to challenge the work of (Saint!) Schuknecht and he was not even an academic. In the 1980s, he was regarded as rather a figure of fun and mocked repeatedly because of instruction courses he delivered at the AAO-HNS meetings. During these demonstrations of a course of treatment for BPPV based on his model of canalolithiasis, he used to use a massage vibrator over the mastoid process (the bump on the temporal bone behind the ear). The attendees responded less-than-professionally, ridiculing him and heaping scorn on him. But don't be sad, dear reader; like most underdogs, Epley had the last laugh. His name is written in medical history in dazzling letters (well, that's how I always picture them), and his canalith repositioning maneuver (CRP)[137]—

135 Çakir BÖ, Ercan İ, Çakir ZA, Civelek Ş, Sayin İ, Turgut S. (2006) What Is the True Incidence of Horizontal Semicircular Canal Benign Paroxysmal Positional Vertigo? *Otolaryngology–Head and Neck Surgery*. 2006;134(3):451-454. https://doi.org/10.1016/j.otohns.2005.07.045.

136 Prokopakis, E; Vlastos, I.M; Tsagournisakis, M. (2013) Canalith Repositioning Procedures among 965 Patients with Benign Paroxysmal Positional Vertigo. *Audiology & Neurotology*, 01/2013, Volume 18, Issue 2. https://doi.org/10.1159/000343579.

137 Epley J.M. (1992).The Canalith Repositioning Procedure: for treatment of benign paroxysmal positional vertigo. *Otolaryngology-Head and Neck Surgery*, vol. 107, no. 3, pp. 399–404, 1992. https://doi.org/10.1177/019459989210700310.

also known as, you guessed it, the Epley maneuver—a very practical, very ingenious, and absolutely noninvasive technique, is still in use all over the world. Numerous studies have investigated its efficacy, with reports of up to 90% of patients being cured with only one treatment.[138]

Epley initially advised patients to sleep in an upright position, supported by pillows, for two days following a canalith repositioning procedure (CRP). They were also instructed to limit their movements, especially avoiding bending over or looking up, to prevent repositioned particles from dislodging. However, these guidelines have changed over the years.[139] The research on the value of such follow-up precautions is mixed.[140] However, I firmly believe they are worth observing. I used to have my patients use very lightweight but sturdy neck supports following CRP, and nearly 99% of them showed no evidence of residual nystagmus in the first week following treatment.[141]

In 2005, I authored a paper discussing how patients sometimes experience a powerful falling sensation after undergoing the Epley maneuver.[142] This paper marked the first publication on this particular topic. While I cannot definitively say whether it influenced the thoughts of others in the OHNS community or altered the direction of research, it still was a necessary contribution. Why? Firstly, when a patient reports feeling like they are falling after undergoing CRP, it is a strong indicator that the maneuver was effective. I hypothesize that this sensation occurs when small masses of otoconia dislodge and fall into the utricle. Although these crystals originated in the utricle, they now exist as free-floating particles that stimulate

138 Fife TD, Iverson DJ, Lempert T, et al (2008). Practice parameter: therapies for benign paroxysmal positional vertigo (an evidence-based review): report of the quality standards subcommittee of the American Academy of Neurology. *Neurology*. 70(22):2067–2074. DOI: 10.1212/01. wnl.0000313378.77444.ac.

139 Epley (1992).

140 Roberts R. A., Gans R. E., DeBoodt J. L., Lister J. J. (2005). Treatment of benign paroxysmal positional vertigo: the necessity of post maneuver patient restrictions. *Journal of the American Academy of Audiology*. 2005;16(6):357–366. DOI: 10.3766/jaaa.16.6.4.

141 Uneri A. (2005). Falling sensation in patients who undergo the Epley maneuver: a retrospective study. *Ear, Nose & Throat Journal*. 2005. Journals.sagepub.com, https://doi.org/10.1177/014556130508400211.

142 Uneri (2005).

the macula unexpectedly. While it is challenging to confirm, these "falling" episodes bear striking similarities to Tumarkin crises regarding symptoms.

Secondly, and perhaps most importantly, failing to anticipate the possibility of a patient experiencing a fall as a side effect of CRP can lead to unpreparedness on the part of the healthcare provider, potentially resulting in injury to the patient. While the risk of a patient falling after CRP is low, anyone administering CRP should be cognizant of this possibility and ready to address it. I first became aware of this potential side effect of CRP during my initial year of performing the maneuver at MUNSI. Taking precautionary measures, we had our patients wear Frenzel goggles (quirky yet practical, functional, and cost-effective) during their CRP. These goggles allowed us to monitor patients' downbeat nystagmus if they reported a powerful and frightening sensation of falling. Following a couple of rather startling experiences, I modified our CRP protocol. We started securely holding our patients during the final stage of the maneuver to ensure their safety.

Benign paroxysmal positional vertigo is commonly accepted as a mechanical problem restricted to the inner ear. Usually, it is summarized as follows: otoconia dislodge; positional vertigo starts; sometimes we find or suspect some kind of triggers such as head trauma or viral infection, but usually, we have no idea why it happens or recurs or whether we can prevent its occurrence. The main diagnostic criteria for BPPV are the same as those for similar vertigo syndromes: the presence of nystagmus associated with some degree of vertigo evoked by positional changes of the head. In short, its diagnosis is symptomatic only. Making a diagnosis based only on symptoms isn't a problem in itself. Still, limiting our understanding to the inner ear alone and neglecting the patient as a "whole being" presents a significant impediment.

According to a 2017 posting on the AAO-HNS website, "a primary complaint of dizziness accounts for an estimated 5.6 million clinic visits in the United States per year, and between 17 and 42 percent of patients (which translates to between 952,000 and 2,352,000 patients) with vertigo ultimately receive a diagnosis of BPPV." It's crucial to identify and understand what is causing these episodes to prevent them from happening and, more importantly, prevent residual dizziness.[143]

Also, there is an alarming statement on the AAO-HNS website, which asserts that "BPPV is very common, and most cases of BPPV happen for no reason." While the specific cause may elude us, it is imperative to recognize that there must be underlying factors contributing to these episodes. Understanding these reasons is necessary for preventing their occurrence and recurrence and mitigating residual dizziness. The statement continues; "Nearly 86 percent of individuals with BPPV report disruptions to their daily activities, leading to lost workdays. Among them, 68 percent reduced their workload, 4 percent changed their jobs, and 6 percent quit their jobs due to the condition. BPPV is more prevalent among older individuals, significantly impacting their health and quality of life. Older patients with BPPV are at a higher risk of falls, depression, and limitations in daily activities. The diagnosis of BPPV is estimated to cost approximately $2,000 per patient, with over 65 percent undergoing potentially unnecessary diagnostic testing or therapeutic interventions. The healthcare costs associated with diagnosing BPPV alone reach $2 billion annually."[144]

The main reason for this challenge lies in our need to improve how we address it. Consider, for instance, the case of some BPPV patients who continue to experience residual dizziness even after a successful canalith repositioning procedure (CRP). Despite the general wealth of literature on vertigo, there is a glaring absence of information on managing residual dizziness following successful CRPs. There is little surprise by this gap, given the challenges medical practitioners face to provide comprehensive follow-up care for their vertigo patients.

143 M. Von Brevern, A. Radtke, A. H. Clarke, and T. Lempert. (2004). "Migrainous vertigo presenting as episodic positional vertigo," *Neurology*, vol. 62, no. 3, pp. 469–472, 2004. DOI: https://doi.org/10.1212/01.

144 Bhattacharyya, N., Gubbels, S. P., Schwartz, S. R., Edlow, J. A., El-Kashlan, H., Fife, T., Holmberg, J. M., Mahoney, K., Hollingsworth, D. B., Roberts, R., Seidman, M. D., Steiner, R. W., Do, B. T., Voelker, C. C., Waguespack, R. W., Corrigan, M. D. (2017). Clinical Practice Guideline: Benign Paroxysmal Positional Vertigo (Update). *Otolaryngol–Head and Neck Surgery*, 2017 Mar; 156 (3_suppl):S1-S47. DOI: 10.1177/0194599816689667.

Imagine the disappointment felt by a healthcare professional encountering a dizzy patient during a follow-up visit after performing what they believed to be a flawless CRP. Naturally, one expects to see a healed, satisfied, and content patient during follow-up examinations. However, when confronted with continuing dizziness post-CRP, most professionals tend to resort to conventional methods like vestibular suppressants or antidepressants. While some may recommend vestibular exercises, these interventions often fall short of resolving the problem.

Residual dizziness following successful CRPs is far more prevalent than existing literature suggests. It can persist for weeks, months, or even years, and for some patients, it proves to be even more distressing than their original episode of BPPV.[145]

Convicted of living with an unsolved "dizziness problem," many patients develop anxiety or depression, which, of course, brings its own challenges. Still, many controversies and arguments are going on about the etiology, classification, and understanding of BPPV, the same as for other vestibular disorders; consequently, complete understanding and treatment of the RD after successful CRP is still on hold.

Another challenge to understanding and treating residual dizziness after successful CRP is that there is still much controversy and disagreement about the etiology and classification of both BPPV and other vestibular disorders. Until there is a shared understanding of these disorders among the medical community it will be nigh on impossible to establish a reliable course of care.

One way we could better understand peripheral vestibular disorders is through taking a holistic perspective. The challenge is to perceive the peripheral vestibular system as operating independently within the patient and attribute the source of vestibular problems exclusively to vestibular

---

145 De Stefano A., Dispenza F. (2017). Understanding Benign Paroxysmal Positional Vertigo. Jaypee Brothers Medical Publishers, Pvt Ltd; Illustrated edition (February 6, 2017). ISBN:9789385999055, 9385999052.

organs. This approach aims to isolate the vestibular system from the broader nervous system and locate the etiology solely within the inner ear.

Another hurdle is that much of the current disagreement about classifications and possible treatments can be traced back to short follow-up periods. Patients are tracked for only a short time, a couple of weeks at best. My own experience as a practitioner showed me that if we can follow up with patients long enough—that is, over at least a couple of years —we will likely see those patients present many other forms of vestibular problems over time.

I'm not alone in this belief; Michael Paparella followed up with his vertigo patients for several years and later wrote, "While obtaining very careful histories from Meniere disease patients over the years, we have found that BPPV is a common concomitant condition. For example, when a patient with vertigo has a 'bad vestibular day,' motion may trigger or exacerbate a prolonged vertiginous spell. In addition, based on our study of 500 patients with Meniere disease, we estimate that approximately 65% to 70% of patients will experience BPPV between episodes of Meniere disease. Therefore, canalith repositioning procedures are sometimes beneficial for Meniere disease patients in addition to other forms of medical management."[146]

When you look at the literature, it might seem there has been a huge awakening at first glance, but some confusion still reigns. Depending on which study you read, BPPV, Meniere's disease, and migraine coincidence vary from 0.3% to 70%, which is a shocking variation. But in some ways, it also sums up the state of current knowledge about vertigo. We know that BPPV is the second-most-common vertigo diagnosis and is almost accepted as a simple mechanical issue—that is, the inner ear crystals are spilling—but we don't know why it happens. We also know that it tends to recur, and sometimes patients end up with prolonged or worse chronic

---

146 Paparella M.M. (2008). Benign paroxysmal positional vertigo and other vestibular symptoms in Meniere disease. *Ear, Nose and Throat Journal* (Vol. 87, Issue 10). DOI: 10.1177/014556130808701006.

dizziness—but we don't know why that happens either. I pick up on these points and my thoughts about them in Chapter 8, but in the meantime, I hope I've given you enough to make you wonder if maybe these disorders are tied together by a common thread.

Did Mr. F.P.'s Crystals Return to Their Nest?

One beautiful spring morning, Ms. R.P., an experienced nurse who had worked at one of the big university hospitals in Istanbul for nearly twenty years, phoned me on behalf of her father, a sixty-two-year-old retired elementary school teacher. A year ago, he had a sudden and severe episode of vertigo one night after dinner. He fell off his chair and subsequently experienced nausea, vomiting, and severe imbalance; he never lost consciousness. He was immediately taken to the neurology clinic of the hospital where his daughter worked and was diagnosed with a probable stroke. However, his MRIs showed no ischemic or hemorrhagic stroke damage, and other diagnostic tests were normal as well. His severe vertigo subsided in two weeks, but his balance did not return to normal. The neurology clinic diagnosed him with a transient ischemic episode, commonly known as a mini-stroke, and referred him to physical therapy (PT) for rehabilitation. However, a year after his stroke and PT, he was still unable to walk without help and relied on a walker to counteract his balance problems.

Miss R.P. brought her father to our clinic to get our opinion about his condition.

"How do you feel?" I asked him.

"Completely normal if I don't stand up," he answered with a wry smile. "I was so excited about my retirement and hoping to have a wonderful time after working for so long, and then this happened."

I wished I could help him, but having read his clinical history, I wasn't optimistic. However, I gave him a routine OHNS examination and, with my assistant, led him to an examination bed to perform the Dix-Hallpike test. Much to our mutual surprise and his evident distress, he experienced very strong left posterior canal nystagmus. I calmed him down and applied an Epley maneuver. After the maneuver, he had an extreme sensation of falling. A couple of minutes later, we let him step down from the bed; he stood, checked himself, and took a few small steps. We stood near him with our arms outstretched and ready to catch him should he stumble, but he walked back to the office without any help. If I had not seen this with my own eyes, I would have been skeptical, to say the very least.

A week later, Ms. R.P. brought her father back for a follow-up examination. It was incredible: he was completely normal; there was no nystagmus during the Dix-Hallpike test and no sign of any imbalance. Even today, I find myself wondering about his first medical episode. Did he really have a minor stroke, and his BPPV was unrelated to it, or did he have a pure vestibular episode, probably a Tumarkin crisis (regarding the fall from the chair) with a resultant BPPV? I suspect I will never know for sure. But one thing I do know is that this is one of my favorite BPPV success stories.

CHAPTER 7

WHERE DOES MIGRAINE COME INTO ALL OF THIS?

Presumably, migraines and, consequently, vertigo are as old as human history, but we can't say that their correlation is as well-known as their suffering natures.

There is not much information about how Sumerians dealt with migraines, but Dr. Walter Alvarez wrote in 1963, "I am satisfied that men have suffered migraine ever since the dawn of written history."[147] The cause of his satisfaction depended on his own discovery in a Sumerian poem/inscription written 5,000 years ago. The poem was about Enki and Ninhursag and said:

> The sick eyed says not
>
> I am sick eyed.
>
> The sick headed (says) not
>
> I am sick headed.

---

147 WC Alvarez, Headache. Notes on the history of migraine. *The Journal of Head and Face Pain*, 1963.

Alvarez wrote, "I can easily imagine a migrainous poet writing 5.000 years ago, and looking forward to a time when he would no longer have to suffer from his blinding headaches." Alvarez continued with another Mesopotamian poem, which was found by his friend, Dr. Sigerist;

> The head throbs,
>
> When pain smites the eyes
>
> And vision dimmed

According to Alvarez, "This certainly is a perfect description of a spell of migraine." I don't know your thoughts, but I am convinced.

If we start with Egyptian physicians,[148] at least in four well-known medical papyri mentioned "half of the head" or "one side of the head" headaches: Ebers, Beatty, Leiden, and Deir El Medina. Sadly other symptoms of a migraine, which is used to call a headache a "migraine headache," were not indicated in these papyri. Only Ebers wrote "spitting mouth" twice with headache, and maybe mentioning "vomiting," but it is impossible to be sure.[149]

Let's explore the wisdom of the father of physicians, Hippocrates.[150] In his own words, he perfectly described a migraine headache, perhaps detailing an exact crisis of one of his patients: "He seemed to see something shining before him like a light, usually in the part of the right eye; at the end of a moment, a violent pain supervened in the right temple, then in all the head and neck... vomiting, when it became possible, was able to divert the pain and render it more moderate." This description encompasses three main elements of a typical migraine headache: visual aura, unilateral headache, and vomiting with an easing of the pain. Hippocrates possessed a wealth of experience and understanding. Additionally, he was an early advocate

---

148 Karenberg, A; Leitz, C. Headache in magical and medical papyri of Ancient Egypt *Cephalalgia*, 11/2001, Volume 21, Issue 9.

149 Søren Ventegodt, Comparison of the medical principles of the ancient Egyptian and the ancient Greek medicine based on the medical papyri... *Journal of Alternative Medicine Research*, 04/2020, Volume 12, Issue 2.

150 Jones WHS. *Hippocrates*. Vol. I–IV. London: William Heinemann, 1923-1931.

of drug therapy and, to my amazement and awe, mentioned the hellebore family of plants for their diuretic action.

We are still determining whether Sumerians or Egyptians recognized the association between migraine and vertigo, and even Hippocrates' understanding of the correlation still needs to be discovered. However, Aretaeus' writings on migraine have come down to us, demonstrating his superb knowledge that migraine and vertigo/dizziness are closely related.

Now it is time to meet with the "prodigy man" of migraine. Among all the ancient authors, Aretaeus[151] holds particular importance; his writings have been referenced by many physicians for centuries. His headache classification aligns remarkably with our current understanding. It wouldn't be far-fetched to claim that the roots of the present subdivision into tension-type headache and migraine may be traced back to Aretaeus' work.

Aretaeus, born in Cappadocia, Asia Minor (present-day Turkey), likely in the early second century, remains somewhat of an enigma in terms of his life. It is believed that he pursued studies in Alexandria, practiced in Rome, and was associated with the eclectic school of thought.

Only two of his works survived, one on pathology (De causis et signis acutorum et chronicorum morborum) and the other on therapy (De therapia acutorum et chronicorum morborum), but we know from the references in these two works that he wrote on numerous other subjects such as fever, surgery, and drugs; unfortunately, they all perished. His works in Greek were unknown until Junius Paulus Crassus (Venice, 1552) translated them into Latin. Latin translations of his two writings were published as eight books (four for each work).[152] He described many nervous and mental disorders, presenting genuine and masterful descriptions of these diseases. Herman Boerhaave (1668–1738), considered the founder of clinical teaching and modern academic hospitals, frequently referred to Aretaeus in his "Praelectiones." He refers to Aretaeus repeatedly in the vertigo chapter, in

151 Pearce JM. The Neurology of Aretaeus: Radix Pedis Neurologia. *Eur Neurol.* 2013;70(1-2):106-12.

152 Koehler P.J., van de Wiel T.W.M., Aretaeus on Migraine and Headache. *The Netherlands Journal of the History of the Neurosciences.* 2001, Vol. 10, No. 3, pp. 253±261.

which Boerhaave acknowledged Aretaeus, noting "he mentioned head-ache as one of the precursors of vertigo..."

Aretaeus' work translated from Greek to English first by Moffat (1785) and succeeded by Francis Adams's versions (1856).

The following paragraph is a one-to-one translation of Arateaus from his Chapter III on Vertigo, or Scotoma.[153] "If darkness possesses the eyes, and if the head be whirled round with dizziness, and the ears ring as from the sound of rivers rolling along with a great noise, or like the wind when it roars among the sails, or like the clang of pipes or reeds, or like the rattling of a carriage..." He continues, "We refer to this condition as vertigo, which can be quite troublesome whether it emerges as a symptom of a head issue, follows from a headache, or presents independently as a chronic illness...The vertigo experience includes a feeling of heaviness in the head, accompanied by flashes of light in the eyes amid significant darkness and a sense of disori-entation towards oneself and the surroundings. In severe cases, individuals may feel weakness in their limbs, leading to a sensation of crawling on the ground, coupled with feelings of nausea and vomiting ..."[154]

It's highly probable that Aretaeus' writings and theories influenced Meniere's work. At one point, Meniere proposed a possible etiology of migraines related to the inner ear, stating, "I do not hesitate to regard these migraines as dependent upon a lesion of the inner ear; they are accompa-nied by noises, by vertigo, by gradual diminution of hearing..."[155]

Meniere further described migraine headaches as the fourth symptom in his original 1861 papers, noting their repeated presence in patients with vertigo, tinnitus, and hearing loss, and he proposed a common etiology between migraine headaches and the symptomatic triad of Meniere's dis-ease. He argued whether the presence of migraine headaches was negligible or suggestive of a clinically significant pattern in his patients. Additionally,

---

153 Francis A. LL.D. *The Extant Works of Aretaeus, The Cappadocian.* By Aretaeus. (trans.). Boston, Milford House, 1972 (Republication of the 1856 edition).

154 Francis A. LL.D. (1972)

155 Baloh R. Prosper Ménière and His Disease. *Arch Neurol.* 2001;58(7):1151–1156.

he suggested that the consistent presentation of migraine headaches in his patients made them unlikely to be comorbidities; instead, he regarded them as a unique component of the syndrome, later coined Meniere's disease, with all symptoms sharing a common etiology.

In 1864, a new medical journal named "Archiv für Ohrenheilkunde" dedicated to otology began publishing,[156] with Anton von Tröltsch, Adam Politzer, and Hermann Schwartze as editors. Tröltsch, Schwartze, and Arnold Pagenstechehey wrote multiple articles referencing headaches and recurrent vertigo in various frameworks.[157]

Meniere may have influenced his contemporaries, as indicated by Adam Politzer's visit to him, documented in their biographies.[158-159]

However, when Politzer described Meniere's disease five years after Meniere's death, he didn't mention headaches in his description of vertigo. In the same year, August Lucae[160] referenced Politzer when describing a patient with Meniere's disease, including headaches as a symptom.

In 1873, Lieving[161] assigned a chapter to vertigo in his masterpiece, "On megrim, sick-headache and some allied disorders: A Contribution to the Pathology of Nerve-storms." Lieving acknowledged the link of migraine (he called it megrim) and vertigo, stating "We already have seen that the phenomena of the megrim-paroxysm are almost exclusively sensory; that the various senses are successively involved, giving rise to blindness and ocular spectra, to numbness and tingling, to subjective tastes and sounds

---

156 Legent F, Gourevitch D, Verry E, Morgon AH, Michel O. Prosper Menière, auriste et érudit. 1799–1862. Paris: Flammarion; 1999.

157 Moshtaghi O., Sahyouni R., Lin H.W., Ghavami Y., and Djalilian H.R. A Historical Recount: Discovering Menière's Disease and its Association with Migraine Headaches. *Otol Neurotol.* 2016 September; 37(8): 1199–1203.

158 Mudry A. The role of Adam Politzer (1835–1920) in the history of otology. *Am J Otol.* 2000;21(5):753–63.

159 Politzer A. Ueber Laesion des Labyrinthes. *Arch Ohrenheil.* 1867;2:88–99.

160 Lucae A. Ohrenkrankheiten. Jahresbericht Über die Leistungen und Fortschritte in ser Gesammten Medicin. 1867;2:455–463.

161 Lieving E., *On Megrim, Sick Headache and Some Allied Disorders. A Contribution to the Pathology of Nerve Storms.*. "The next feature of the paroxysm which requires our notice is giddiness or vertigo" (page 121),1873, London.

and to acute pain. It need not, then, surprise us to find the muscular sense also sometimes sharing the disorder and giving rise to various degrees of vertiginous sensation. A certain sense of giddiness is, in fact, incidental to the progress of the seizure (Migraine episode) in many cases, and I see that it was particularly noticed by ten of the patients whose cases I have collected in the table. Sometimes it is accompanied with great nausea and is increased by every attempt to rise or move, constituting a condition, not unlike the first stage of sea-sickness, and, like it, maybe relieved by actual vomiting. As a rule, it occurs after the disorders of sight, touch, and speech, when these form a part of the seizure, and either attend or follow the development of the headache." He continues; "The giddiness of megrim to which I have just referred (unless, perhaps, in the last-mentioned cases, of which we have no particulars) chiefly affects the general sense of equilibrium, and is not attended with any apparent rotatory or other movements of visual images of a very striking character. There is, however, another distressing form of vertigo sometimes associated with megrim, in which these visual phenomena are highly developed and constitute a principal part of the seizure (Migraine episode). This I have known to occur, if not in the course of the ordinary megrim paroxysm, yet intercurrently, and probably vicariously with it."

In summary, despite Meniere's initial proposition that migraine headaches are linked to the classical triad of symptoms—tinnitus, vertigo, and hearing loss—and Lieving's classic *Migraine* textbook, which acknowledged the connection between vertigo and migraine, these ideas did not gain widespread approval in medical society.

In the present day, Meniere's disease is clinically diagnosed based on the AAO-HNS criteria, while migraine is diagnosed according to the International Headache Society (IHS). Notably, only the IHS provides diagnostic criteria for vestibular migraine independently from AAO-HNS.[162]

---

162 Jose A. Lopez-Escamez, John Carey, Won-Ho Chung, Joel A. Goebel, Måns Magnusson, Marco Mandalà, David E. Newman-Toker, Michael Strupp, Mamoru Suzuki, Franco Trabalzini and Alexandre Bisdorff. Equilibrium Committee Amendment to the 1995 AAO-HNS Guidelines for the Definition of Ménière's Disease. Diagnostic criteria for Ménière's disease. *Journal of Vestibular Research* 25 (2015).

Despite this differentiation, the link between migraine and vertigo has been recognized since the time of Aretaeus. Studies have found that "vestibular migraines" can be present without any headache in 30% of cases, and 45% of patients with Meniere's disease have at least one accompanying migraine symptom.[163],[164]

Is This a Duck or a Rabbit?

The beginning of wisdom is to call things by their proper name.
– Confucius

Like the duck-rabbit illusion, which can be perceived as both a duck and a rabbit simultaneously, the debate surrounding the distinction between migraine and Meniere's disease has persisted since Prosper Meniere's time and continues to be relevant today.[165] In his 1861 series of four papers, Meniere identified vertigo, tinnitus, and hearing loss as a unified symptom group. Surprisingly, he included migraine headaches in this group, attributing them to the exact etiology and origin—the inner ear. Meniere's original proposal suggests that migraine headaches are related to tinnitus, vertigo, and hearing loss, all stemming from the inner ear.

Before we start the discussion, let's clarify: do we truly understand what migraine is?

More than 50 years ago, in 1970, in the first publication of "Migraine," Oliver Sacks wrote, "The chief features of migraine—its phenomena, and how these are experienced by the patient, its mode of occurrence, the triggers that may provoke it, the general ways in which one may live with it

163 Radtke A, Lempert T, Gresty MA, Brookes GB, Bronstein AM, Neuhauser H. Migraine and Ménière's disease: is there a link? *Neurology.* 2002;59(11):1700–4.

164 Ghavami Y, Mahboubi H, Yau AY, Maducdoc M, Djalilian HR. Migraine features in patients with Ménière's disease. *Laryngoscope.* 2015.

165 Chen, JY., Guo, ZQ., Wang, J. et al. Vestibular migraine or Meniere's disease: a diagnostic dilemma. *J Neurol.* 270, 1955–1968 (2023). https://doi.org/10.1007/s00415-022-11532-x

or combat it—none of this has changed in 2000 years. Thus, a vivid and detailed description of these matters is always relevant and cannot become obsolete." He continues, "Migraine affects a substantial minority of the population, occurs in all civilizations, and has been recognized since the dawn of recorded history. If it was a scourge or an encouragement to Caesar, Paul, Kant, and Freud, it is also a daily fact of life to anonymous millions who suffer in secrecy and silence. Its nature and causes puzzled Hippocrates and have been the subject of argument for two thousand years." It is hard to believe, but it is still more puzzling and contentious than ever.

In 1999, Dieterich and Brandt[166] presented retrospective research. "Episodic vertigo related to migraine (90 cases): vestibular migraine?" However, there was trouble: "Since most of the patients (n = 83) did not fulfill the HIS criteria for basilar migraine but could be cured by medical migraine treatment, diagnosis of episodic vertigo or dizziness related to migraine was based, first, on the history of at least five episodes in which vertigo or dizziness was a major complaint in any period of time, and second, on one of the following four typical groups (A–D) into which the response to migraine treatment was included." As you can see, there is trouble because most of their patients did not meet the criteria for basilar migraine according to established guidelines, yet they responded well to migraine treatment. As a result, they decided that their diagnosis of episodic vertigo or dizziness related to migraine was based on specific criteria, including a history of at least five episodes of vertigo or dizziness and a positive response to migraine treatment. However, the discrepancy between patients' symptoms and established diagnostic criteria posed a challenge in accurately defining and diagnosing their condition.

Here is the Brandt and Dietrich's Vestibular Migraine algorithm.[167]

---

166 Brandt T., Dieterich M. Episodic vertigo related to migraine (90 cases): vestibular migraine? *J Neurol.* 1999; 246: 883-892.

167 Brandt T., Dieterich M., 1999.

Alev Uneri

Group A

- Recurrent episodes of vertigo or dizziness and nonvestibular neurological deficits attributable to a dysfunction in the brainstem.
- Associated headache during or immediately after vertigo or dizziness ("brainstem aura with headache").
- Individual history of migraine.

Group B

- Recurrent episodes of vestibular and/or ocular motor dysfunction only.
- Associated headache during or immediately after vertigo/dizziness ("only vestibular or ocular motor aura with headache").
- Individual history of migraine.

Group C

- Recurrent episodes of vestibular and/or ocular motor dysfunction only.
- Associated headache during or immediately after vertigo dizziness ("only vestibular or ocular motor aura with headache").
- Efficacy of medical (migraine) treatment.

Group D

- Recurrent episodes of vestibular and/or ocular motor dysfunction only.

- Without associated headache during or immediately after vertigo dizziness ("only vestibular or ocular motor aura with headache")

- Efficacy of medical (migraine) treatment

Brandt and Dietrich also wrote, "These categories allowed us to define constellations based on the minimal features necessary to assess the diagnosis. All our patients showed the features of at least one of these constellations. Many presented with features of more than one category, especially when observed over a longer time."

As you can see, to address the challenge posed by the "migraine criteria fulfillment of IHS," they had to create another classification. However, this also means that if you had only four episodes, you had to wait until your fifth episode to receive an accurate diagnosis. Despite sounding somewhat absurd, the reality is that most physicians have to adhere to a particular classification. I want to finish this chapter with a quotation from Amit Goswami, who wrote, "Science, you see, proceeds by a very fundamental assumption of the way things are or must be" (from "The Self-Aware Universe," 1995).

CHAPTER 8

MY EUREKA MOMENT

To convince someone of the truth, it is not enough to state it,
but rather one must find the path from error to truth.
– Wittgenstein

Have you ever found yourself agreeing to something you know will be tedious? Maybe it's because of friendship, difficulty saying no, or even a well-placed bribe like a box of donuts. In 2000, I found myself in precisely that situation.

It was my fourth year with the Institute. By that point, it's fair to say we were victims of our own success. We were accepting too many patients, our schedules were bursting at the seams, and I was struggling with the classification paper, which seemed increasingly unachievable. On one particularly hectic day, Dr. Dilsad Turkdogan, who ran the pediatric neurology unit two floors above mine, visited my office. She explained that she was planning to write an article about pediatric migraine cases and asked if I could conduct vestibular tests on her patients. Vestibular tests are time-consuming, which makes them challenging for the person conducting them. However, this is nothing compared to the challenge they present for the person on the receiving end, particularly if the test is an electro-nystagmography (ENG). During an ENG, electrodes are attached near the eyes to record eye movements, while warm and cold water or air (7 degrees Celsius colder or warmer than body temperature) stimulates the inner ear. If the inner ear is healthy, the eyes will move involuntarily (nystagmus), and the recorded response will be the same degree in both ears.

It's a painless test, but if you have a healthy and fully working vestibular system, it causes you to experience vertigo. You'll probably feel nauseous, and you might even vomit. Having an ENG is really not something you're likely to have on your bucket list. Furthermore, conducting an ENG—especially on kids—was certainly not at the top of my wish list. However, as I'm sure you've guessed, I said yes. I did it for the sake of scientific curiosity (and a bit of reluctance to say no—and yes, yes, perhaps the offer of donuts played a little role, too).

To this day, I am grateful I did not say no. The experience changed my perspective on vertigo entirely. I realized not only that migraine and vestibular syndromes are strongly intertwined but also that kids are just as susceptible to these syndromes as adults are. And bonus, the research paper was published in 2003.[168]

While examining and testing children who experienced migraines, I engaged in conversations with their mothers. Over time, I realized that these conversations yielded crucial information that might not have surfaced otherwise. One revelation was that many of the mothers were not unfamiliar with dizziness; they had experienced dizziness, migraine headaches, or both in the past. Extracting a history of dizziness was sometimes challenging. Often, individuals who have experienced vertigo do not recognize it as such. When asked about past experiences, they might recall incidents like "food poisoning" that made them "dizzy" and caused vomiting. Still, they were adamant that it wasn't a vertigo episode because it was attributed to food poisoning. Alternatively, they may

168 Uneri A., Turkdogan D. (2003.) Evaluation of vestibular functions in children with vertigo episodes. *Archives of Disease in Childhood*.88(6), 510-511, DOI: 10.1136/adc.88.6.510.

Alev Uneri

recall a viral illness causing "dizziness," dismissing it as insignificant. Perhaps most concerning is when individuals attribute their episodes of dizziness" or chronic dizziness to psychological factors due to a previous diagnosis. These examples highlight the misconception that "vertigo" is a distinct condition, not a symptom, leading many to perceive "dizziness" and "vertigo" as separate entities.

Working with these children and their families brought about a fleeting moment of what I would call Ionian Enchantment. Coined by physician and historian Gerald Holton, Ionian Enchantment refers to a belief in the unity of the sciences. This concept traces back to Thales of Miletus, Ionia, who believed that all matter ultimately consisted of water, reflecting a desire for a unified theory of everything. (This notion continues to prevail in scientific thought today, with figures like Albert Einstein embodying it to the core.[169] Albert Einstein was a true believer in the concept of Grand Unification in physics, and he tried to prove it until his last breath (literally).) As I pieced together the information gleaned from conversations with the mothers, I began to contemplate whether some "vertigo syndromes" could actually be different facets of a single disorder—migraine. While not applicable to all vertigo cases, it is plausible that many peripheral "vertigo syndromes" represent various manifestations of an underlying migraine infrastructure.

Imagine it like looking through a glass prism; when a bright sunbeam shines on it, you can see all the different colors that it contains. Or so you think. In reality, while the colors look different, they are only the components of the light itself.

Oliver Sacks wrote that he had a similar enlightening revelation with his migraine patients: "When I saw my first migraine patient, I thought of migraine as a peculiar type of headache, no more and no less. As I saw more patients, it became apparent to me that headache was never the sole feature of a migraine and, later still, that it was not even a necessary feature of all migraines. I was moved, therefore, to enquire further into a

---

169 Wilson E. O. (1999). *Consilience: The Unity of Knowledge* (reprint). Vintage.

subject which appeared to retreat before me, growing more complex, less capable of circumscription, and less intelligible; the more I learned of it, I delved into the literature of the subject, submerged, and re-emerged, more knowledgeable in some ways but more confused in others. I returned to my patients, whom I found more instructive than any book. And after I had seen a thousand migraine patients, I saw the subject made sense."[170]

Sack's conclusion was pivotal; I immersed myself in the extant literature and emerged more knowledgeable in some ways and more confused in others. By that career stage, I had seen thousands of patients. I revisited my old patients' files and listened with a different perspective to my newer ones. Those patients, essentially my sample group, were incredibly instructive; as I reviewed my notes on their files, things started to fall into place for me. That is not to say that everything suddenly became clear; I was consistently confused, baffled, and intrigued as I saw the same patient presenting with "different" clinical features at various times. For example, one patient whom I successfully treated for vertigo, aural fullness, and fluctuant sensorineural hearing loss in low frequencies, all of which were recorded as being due to Meniere's disease, came to see me eighteen months later with benign paroxysmal positional vertigo (BPPV). I successfully treated him with a canalith repositioning procedure (CRP), only to see him again six months later when he was experiencing prolonged dizziness. While not all patients showed this series of symptoms, many did—enough, in fact, to suggest that there was a pattern, irregular maybe, but still a pattern. I realized that if healthcare professionals have the chance to follow up with their patients over time—and by that, I mean years—a very different picture will emerge than the one we create from looking only at a patient's immediate situation.

Hippocrates wrote, "It is far more important to know what person the disease has than what disease the person has." While the "Our Clinic's Vertigo Patients Classification Paper" remained unwritten, I did learn to understand my dizzy patients.

---

170 Sacks, O. (1970). *Migraine*. Preface to the original (1970) edition. University of California Press.

Alev Uneri

Finding Time: A Doctor's Crusade for Patient Connection

I joined MUNSI at its inception, establishing Turkey's first dedicated vertigo and dizziness clinic amid modest funding and significant debt.

Despite preexisting vestibular research labs in several major university hospital OHNS departments, this clinic marked the country's first specialized facility for dizzy patients. Notably, the OHNS department at Hacettepe University in Ankara housed one such lab, primarily focusing on diagnostics since the 1970s. During my residency, mandatory rotations in the vestibular clinic provided invaluable training in ENG and audiometry exams. It was a pioneering OHNS clinic during the 1980s.

Patient outreach took time, with initial months seeing only a handful of patients. However, this allowed ample time—unprecedented in my career— to devote to each patient. With an average of twelve patients weekly, I dedicated approximately two hours to each appointment. Conducting thorough personal health histories, OHNS examinations, and utilizing Frenzel goggles for nystagmus assessment were routine. Audiometry tests supplemented our evaluations, guiding further diagnostic steps like ENG or CDP if needed. Fortunately, by the time patients reached us, they had typically undergone a battery of basic tests to eliminate other potential causes of their vertigo, such as neurological conditions, which helped to save time in creating a diagnosis.

I quickly realized the importance of encouraging patients to share not only their immediate symptoms but also other aspects of their health histories and lifestyles. These conversations often revealed valuable "snippets" of information, such as motion sickness in the past, the tendency for hypotension, a propensity for headaches, irritable bowel syndrome (IBS), or a vertigo episode misdiagnosed as food poisoning (or some other verdict) years ago. Each piece of information was like a puzzle piece, helping me form a clearer picture of the patient's problem. Collecting and assembling these "snippets" painted a clearer picture of what was going on, aiding accurate diagnosis and tailored treatment plans.

As patient numbers grew, maintaining this comprehensive approach became challenging. I refused to compromise by rushing appointments or overbooking, even as my waitlist stretched to months. However, this dedication came at a cost, as the demands took their toll and led to burnout. Eventually, after eleven years, I made the difficult decision to leave the clinic.

Vertigo Chronicles: My First Encounter with Sir Vertigo von Nystagmus

The otolaryngologist Jeremy Hornibrook[171] quotes Shakespeare's Romeo and Juliet in one of his papers. Specifically, in Act I, Scene II, Bevolio says, "Tut man, one fire burns out another's burning. One pain is lessen'd by another's anguish; turn giddy, and be holp by backwards turning...." I strongly suspect Shakespeare himself suffered from vertigo. How else could he empathize so closely with someone who experienced it?

I had my own moment of Shakespearean empathy when I experienced my first fully fledged vestibular episode. I was in my forties, and it happened when I was on vacation in a beautiful resort in Antalya in late summer. I was so tired from work and happy to be on vacation and finally relax. I love swimming, and swimming in the Mediterranean Sea in late summer is heaven as far as I'm concerned. The water is warm and very calm, especially in the early mornings. On the first day of our vacation, while I was swimming in the sea before breakfast, a whack of motion sickness hit me out of nowhere. I was far from the shore. As I turned to swim back to shore, almost overcome with nausea, I tried to understand why I was feeling this way. I remember wondering if a large ship was somewhere off in the distance and if its wake had triggered my motion sickness. It seemed plausible at the time. Unfortunately, I was wrong. When I finally reached the beach, I lay in a lounge chair, waiting for the motion sickness to pass. As I lay there, I looked up at the sky. The clouds were bouncing!!! They

---

171 Hornibrook (2011).

were sliding slowly to the left, then jumping back to the right, over and over again. The reality hit me, "Oh my God, I have NYSTAGMUS!" I was having my first vertigo episode. It devoured three days of my one week of leisure, but it could have been much worse. At least I didn't vomit, and I could walk around after the second day. Along with I had the chance to experience a vertigo episode first-hand, which could surely only be helpful in terms of my career.

I had no idea at that point that I had migraine base. To this day, I can't recall ever having what might be described as a "typical" migraine headache. But I did remember that I once had a migraine scotoma—a type of visual aura—without a headache or vertigo. It was kind of a scary experience. I was in an airplane, waiting for takeoff. Suddenly, a brilliant radiance appeared in my left visual field. It took the form of a giant crescent with zigzagged margins fringed with brilliance and spectral colors. It was blindingly bright, and it began to grow wider. I panicked—actually, if I'm being honest, I was already in a state of panic because I had a phobia of flying at that time. But suddenly I remembered something that relieved me. A few months previously, I had read Oliver Sacks' book *Migraine*. Images of the colored scotoma sketches in the book flashed into my mind, and I realized with some relief that this bright "whatever" I was seeing was just like those sketches. "Oh," I thought, "this is an aura, nothing to worry about. No need to panic." Fifteen to twenty minutes after it began, it enlarged, dimmed, filled my left visual field—and then disappeared. I settled down to read my book as if nothing had happened. I didn't even have a headache afterward. You may be wondering whether I discussed my experience with any of my neurology colleagues. Well, I should have done this, of course, but I didn't, because as I said, I'm an MD and in my mind if it wasn't dire, it was nothing important. But I did check *Migraine* (book) as soon as I was home, and my scotoma did indeed match one of the illustrations in the book.

Sacks wrote that "The determinants of migraine are almost infinite in number, and may present themselves in many different combinations."[172]

---

172 Sacks, O. (1995). *Migraine*, p. 117. Picador.

Vestibular migraine is equally diverse in terms of its characteristics. Three-hundred years ago, Thomas Willis, one of the first people to research the anatomy of the brain and nervous system,[173] wrote about migraine determinants: "An evil or weak constitution of parts . . . sometimes innate and hereditary . . . an irritation in some distant member of viscera . . . changes of a season, atmospheric states, the great aspects of sun and moon, violent passions, and errors in diet."[174] I couldn't have put it better myself.

Unmasking the Medical Pretender

By now, you know that I believe that migraine, Meniere's disease, and BPPV are connected and intertwined, and that both my professional experience and the literature support that belief. In fact, researchers and physicians have been writing about the migraine–vertigo correlation since Areteaus' time.[175] Even Prosper Meniere himself pointed out the prevalence of migraine among his vertigo patients,[176] but somehow migraine's and Meniere's disease's etiological paths diverged soon after the good doctor's death. Fortunately, we seem to be coming full circle. You can now find a massive amount of papers about Meniere's disease and its connection with migraine.

In 2004, I authored an article exploring the potential link between benign paroxysmal positional vertigo (BPPV) and migraine.[177] We looked at the records of more than five-hundred patients with BPPV whom we had treated over the years. All of our patients had a confirmed diagnosis of BPPV and were followed for one to seven years. Our retrospective research

173 The Circle of Willis, a circle of arteries on the base of the brain which he described perfectly in his Cerebri Anatome of 1664, is named after him.

174 Pearce J.M.S. (1986). Historical aspects of migraine. *Journal of Neurology, Neurosurgery, and Psychiatry.* 1986;49:1097-1103. doi: 10.1136/jnnp.49.10.1097.

175 Francis Adams L.D. *The Extant Works of Aretaeus, The Cappadocian.* By Aretaeus. (trans.). Boston, Milford House, 1972 (Republication of the 1856 edition).

176 Ménière P; Atkinson M, trans. Gazette Medicale de Paris 1861. Meniere's original papers. *Acta Otolaryngol.* 1961; (suppl 162).

177 Uneri A., Migraine and benign paroxysmal positional vertigo: an outcome study of 476 patients. *Ear, Nose & Throat Journal,* 2004. journals.sagepub.com.

study consisted of detailed patient questionnaires and vestibular tests. The results showed that migraine and motion sickness were three times more common in patients with BPPV than in the general population. Furthermore, a family history of migraine (58.4%) and vertigo (44.9%) was also more common in our patients than in a control group (8% and 24%, respectively.)

Let's practice a little logic exercise: If A is related to B and if A is connected with C, and if B is associated with C, you can easily infer that A, B, and C are related to each other, right? We're in Occam's razor territory now.

Back in 2004, I couldn't find a similar paper to reference while I was writing mine. In mid-2020, I used Google Scholar to search for "BPPV and migraine." My search returned 3,570 results. When I used the search string "Migraine and positional vertigo," I found more than seven-thousand papers. And last but not least, when I used the search string "Meniere's disease and BPPV," it gave me 3,640 results. Out of curiosity, I decided to be less specific and searched for simply "Meniere's disease and positional vertigo." That turned up more than 13,000 results. This is an incredibly significant development. When you continue to dig in the literature, though, you may become bewildered as well as informed, because the figures across the various studies are inconsistent to say the least. For example, in papers where the concomitance rates of BPPV and migraine were discussed, the rates varied from 0.3% to 70%.[178] You don't need a degree in statistics to question the reliability of those figures.

Professor Titus Ibekwe, the National Secretary of the Otorhinolaryngological Society of Nigeria and elected Vice-Chairman of the International Advisory Board (IAB) of the American Academy of Otorhinolaryngology, Head and Neck Surgery Foundation (AAOHNSF),[179] and his team wrote, "There is a statistically significant difference between the prevalence of migraine in

---

178 See Wu, Z. M., Zhang, S. Z., Liu, X. J., Chen, X., Ji, F., Chen, A. T., Yang, W. Y., Han, D. Y. (2007). Benign paroxysmal positioning vertigo related to inner ear disorders. Zhonghua Er Bi Yan Hou Tou Jing Wai Ke Za Zhi 42(11):821–825. PMID: 18300443.

179 Ibekwe, T. S., FasOnla, J. A., Ibekwe, P. U., (2008) Migraine and Meniere's Disease: Two Different Phenomena with Frequently Observed Concomitan. *JAMA*. 100(3).

Meniere's patients and migraine in the overall population (32% vs. 5.3%, $p = 0.001$)" in 2008. For those of you who are not familiar with statistics, especially medical statistics, that shows that migraine in Meniere's disease patients is much more common than in the normal (that is, healthy) population, and strongly suggests a link between the two diseases.

Yet, despite mounting evidence, the medical community's tendency to compartmentalize these conditions persists, often overlooking their underlying unity, so they added another category into the mix: vestibular migraine.

Optimists may view the recognition of vestibular migraine as progress, acknowledging that some vertigo episodes are migraine-related. However, the reality remains that this acknowledgment falls short of addressing the broader spectrum of vertigo disorders.

If healthcare providers recognize that prolonged dizziness, clustered Meniere's episodes, dizziness persisting post-successful CRPs, or frequent BPPV episodes are akin to "migraine equivalents," they can significantly expedite and enhance treatment for chronic vertigo patients. Returning to our earlier reasoning, A (migraine), B (Meniere's), and C (BPPV) are not isolated entities but rather diverse expressions of a singular primary disorder: migraine.

John Godfrey Saxe's Elephant in the Room

Confession time: when it comes to patients with vertigo/dizziness, we, the OHNS and neurology communities, often resemble the six men of Indostan in John Godfrey Saxe's poem "The Blind Men and the Elephant." This fable highlights our tendency as humans to prioritize our limited, subjective experiences over others' when determining the truth of a matter. In our case, the elephant represents migraine. Recognizing the presence of this "elephant" (migraine) allows us to comprehend its various components, which include numerous different vertigo diagnoses like BPPV, Meniere's disease, and other peripheral vertigo diagnoses (such as phobic postural vertigo, psychogenic vertigo bilateral vestibulopathy, vestibular paroxysmia, etc.), all of which are merely different facets of the same underlying entity.

Migraine is one of the most common disorders worldwide, affecting approximately 15%–20% of the adult population in developed countries alone.[180] It is also one of the more common hereditary diseases.[181] Although we still haven't established the exact pattern of inheritance, we know that more than half (nearly three times greater than that of relatives of non-migraineurs) of people who experience migraine have at least one family member who also has migraine headaches.[182]

Once a healthcare provider recognizes that they are dealing with migraine, they can appraise the patient holistically by looking at their genetic background, personal histories, habits, lifestyles, psychology, environment, etc. And once people who suffer from vertigo understand that they are suffering from migraine, they can offer their physician more comprehensive information about their symptoms and other influencing factors. Unfortunately, many vertigo patients continue to suffer because they aren't treated as whole individuals.

This book aims to address this gap. Let me put it another way (if you still need clarification) regarding the migraine as the underlying association. We have known about migraines for nearly two-thousand years and accumulated a vast amount of knowledge about them. First I should admit that we still don't know the exact mechanisms that give rise to a migraine episode or what exactly happens during an episode, but do we know (at least to some degree) how to cope with migraine, how to live with it, and how to minimize the likelihood of triggering an episode.

180 Global Burden of Disease Study 2013 Collaborators. (2015). Global, regional, and national incidence, prevalence, and years lived with disability for 301 acute and chronic diseases and injuries in 188 countries, 1990-2013: a systematic analysis for the Global Burden of Disease Study 2013. *Lancet*, 386(9995). 743-800. DOI: https://doi.org/10.1016/S0140-6736(15)60692-4

181 Stewart, W. F., Staffa, J., Lipton, R. B., Ottman R. (1997) Familial risk of migraine: A population-based study. *Annals of Neurology*.41: 166-172. DOI: 10.1002/ana.410410207.

182 Merikangas, K. R., Risch, N. J., Merikangas, J. R., Weissman, M. M., Kidd, K. K. (1988). Migraine and depression: Association and familial transmission. *Journal of Psychiatric Research*. 22(2), 119-29.

My own experience tells me that people with migraine can be successfully treated, especially by paying attention to their lifestyle choices and habits and being aware of stress factors and even what season it is.

Are you intrigued? I do hope so. Remember, knowledge is power.

Putting My Theory to the Test

Once I realized that many of my patients with peripheral vertigo might actually be experiencing migraine-related symptoms, I set out on a mission to investigate their histories and symptoms. I devised a questionnaire and distributed it to all my peripheral vertigo patients, both new and old, regardless of whether they had consistent complaints or were experiencing new ones.

But before discussing further, let's discuss migraine equivalents. These are also known as migraine auras without headaches or silent migraines, and they encompass a range of neurological symptoms that occur during a migraine attack, minus the headache. Common examples include visual disturbances like flashes of light, blind spots, or zigzag lines. Rarer manifestations may involve sensory changes such as tingling or numbness in the limbs or body, speech difficulties, confusion, and other neurological symptoms. While migraine equivalents are often associated with children, adults can experience them too. In a 2015[183] article, migraine equivalents in children were reported as follows: Motion sickness (42.6%), Limb pain (37.5%), Abdominal migraine (40.4%), Cyclic vomiting (3.7%), and Benign paroxysmal vertigo (8.1%). Interestingly, the authors did not observe any cases of Benign paroxysmal torticollis among their patients, a condition typically seen only in children; however, I encountered an adult female patient with this presentation.

---

183 Tarantino S, De Ranieri C, Dionisi C, Gagliardi V, Capuano A, Vigevano F, Gentile S, Valeriani M. Migraine equivalents and related symptoms, psychological profile and headache features: which relationship? *J Headache Pain*. 2015;16:536. doi: 10.1186/s10194-015-0536-2. Epub 2015 Jun 9. PMID: 26059348; PMCID: PMC4467804.

Alev Uneri

Apart from these well-known equivalents, there are some intriguing and perhaps less recognized symptoms associated with migraines.[184]-[185] These symptoms can often be mistaken for those of a cold or sinus infection and may include fatigue, nasal congestion, sinus pressure, and cognitive symptoms that mimic the feeling of being "foggy" due to a cold. Migraine equivalents are different forms of migraines and can still significantly impact daily functioning, even in the absence of headache pain.

Let's get back to where we left off; I asked four basic questions In the questionnaire:

1. Migraine or equivalents: I asked patients to note any and all types of headaches and equivalents they experienced now and had experienced in the past.

2. Motion sickness: As I noted earlier, people are often unaware that they have suffered from motion sickness unless it was severe, or they think it was simply a childhood thing, and now they are free of it, so it is not worth mentioning. I stressed the importance of thinking about past experiences of motion sickness.

3. Symptoms of irritable bowel syndrome (IBS): Many migraine sufferers have gastrointestinal irregularities (based on my experience with my patients.)

4. Family history:

> A. Have any of their first-degree relative (mother, father, siblings) ever had migraine or migraine equivalents?

> B. Have any of their first-degree relatives (mother, father, siblings) ever had any dizziness, no matter the diagnosis?

In addition to having patients complete the questionnaire, I asked them if their vertigo/dizziness episodes or symptoms were connected with

184 Godley F, Petrarca K. Sinus Migraine: An Emerging Diagnosis. *Pract Pain Manag.* 2022 May/June;22(3).

185 Proctor L.D. Migraine equivalents. Henry Ford Hospital Medical Bulletin. 1960; 8: 4, p. 339.

anything in their daily lives—for example, certain activities, what they ate, etc. My efforts eventually paid off.

As Douglas Adams stated; "I may not have gone where I intended to go, but I think I have ended up where I intended to be." After years of working with vertigo patients and excavating scientific literature, all the information added up, and the curtain went up.

Ladies and Gentlemen, Please Give a Warm Welcome to Vestibular Migraine!

As we have seen, a strong association between vertigo and migraine was established as far back as Aretaeus' time, for at least some researchers.[186] Remember, Aretaeus observed and noted that vertigo episodes were associated with heterocrania (migraine headache), photophobia (a need to avoid light and a desire to seek relief in darkness), visual aura (floating threads in the line of vision), nausea, vomiting, and nystagmus (the eyes move to and fro repeatedly).

It's fair to say the medical community can be a cautious bunch. In this case, they hesitated a little before creating the concept of vestibular migraine. And by "a little," I mean two thousand years. The concept of vestibular migraine was not established until 1999. Moreover, the International Headache Society and Barany Society published consensus criteria for diagnosing vestibular migraine only in . . . 2013 (no rush!).[187] While the current view of vestibular migraine has evolved over the past twenty-five years, progress continues to be slow. Despite millennia of observations and hundreds of articles about the probable association between vestibular symptoms and migraine, there is still no consensus about diagnostic

186 Huppert, D., Brandt, T. (2017). Descriptions of vestibular migraine and Meniere's disease in Greek and Chinese antiquity. *Cephalalgia*. 37:385–390. DOI: 10.1177/0333102416646755.

187 Headache Classification Committee of the International Headache Society (IHS). (2013). The International Classification of Headache Disorders, 3rd edition (beta version). *Cephalalgia*. 33:629–808. DOI: 10.1177/0333102413485658.

criteria or (for some researchers) even the existence of vestibular migraine; instead, disagreement prevails.

As a scientist, I know that the plural of anecdotes is not data, as they say, but the current situation means that millions of patients are not getting the treatment they need. Fortunately, one thing that the medical community in general does agree on is that vestibular migraine is a legitimate neurotologic disorder.

The medical community's struggle to define vestibular migraine is evident in its various attempts to label the disorder. Terms such as Migraine Vestibulopathy, Migrainous Vertigo, Migraine Associated Vertigo (or Migraine-Associated Vertigo), and Vestibular Migraine have all been proposed. Like all my peers, I, too, once wavered between these labels before settling on a preference for Vestibular Migraine (VM), which aligns more closely with the condition and has become the favored term among medical professionals.

However, the debate over terminology pales in comparison to the challenge of obtaining a VM diagnosis, particularly for individuals who have never experienced a classic migraine headache episode, which presents a significant problem because migraine is a complex condition with numerous symptoms that can mimic those of other disorders.

While a migraine sufferer may experience headaches as their primary symptom, these headaches can also be secondary or even absent altogether. The term "migraine equivalent" (or "migraine variant") is used to describe a migraine that presents without a headache. Oliver Sacks wrote: "We justify the use of the term 'migraine equivalent' if the following circumstances are fulfilled: the occurrence of discrete non-cephalgic episodes with a duration, a periodicity, and a clinical format similar to episodes of common migraine, and a tendency to be precipitated by the same type of emotional and physical antecedents."[188]

---

188 Oliver Sacks, *Migraine* (1995), page 34.

Willis and Tissot wrote about people with gastric and ocular migraines in the seventeenth and eighteenth centuries,[189] but it was Edward Liveing who first documented that migraine episodes can come in different forms.[190] His five-hundred-page book *On Megrim, Sick Headache and Some Allied Disorders* is universally accepted as the best text about migraine. In it, he wrote about vertiginous, gastralgic, pectoralgic, asthmatic, epileptic, laryngismal, and maniacal "transformations"' of migraine. Although vertigo as a presentation of migraine had been recognized in the early days of neurology (Liveing, 1873; Escat, 1904; Boenheim, 1917), it took over a century before any systematic studies on the association between vertigo and migraine were published.[191] By this point you may not be surprised to learn that the notion of migraine equivalents has not been broadly or enthusiastically (!) approved yet.

Oliver Sacks wrote, "The physician who presumes to diagnose an 'abdominal migraine' will be regarded, by many of his colleagues, as talking mumbo-jumbo or worse, and it may only be after endless diagnostic investigations and negative laparotomies, or the sudden replacement of episodes of abdominal pain by typical vascular headaches, that the old Victorian term is exhumed and reconsidered."[192]

Although there are growing numbers of peer-reviewed articles on migraine and vertigo and childhood migraine equivalents, we still have a long way to go in terms of understanding and helping vestibular migraine patients, especially those who do not experience headache as part of their migraine.

In 1999, eighty years after the German Felix Boenheim[193] coined the term "vestibular migraine," neurologists Marianne Dieterich and Thomas

189 Pearce, J.M.S. (1986). *Journal of Neurology, Neurosurgery, and Psychiatry.* 49:1097-1103. DOI: 10.1136/jnnp.49.10.1097.

190 Lieving E., (1873)

191 Furman, J., Lempert, T. (2016). Vestibular migraine. *Handbook of Clinical Neurology.* 137, 301-316.

192 Sacks, *Migraine*, p. 35.

193 Boenheim F. (1917) Über familiare hemicrania vestibularis. Neurol Centralbl [need full journal name here]. 36:226–9.

Brandt[194] reintroduced the concept to the medical community. Sort of. However, they used the phrase "migrainous vertigo" instead of vestibular migraine. Dr. Hannelore Neuhaser, an esteemed epidemiologist from the renowned Robert Koch Institute, conducted influential studies on the incidence and prevalence of dizziness (vertigo). Her team also established diagnostic criteria for the condition in 2001.[195]

While diagnostic criteria are essential, it's crucial to remember that vestibular migraine is a complex condition with varied manifestations. Symptoms can differ not only among different patients but also within the same patient at different times. This variability, highlighted in Chapter 4 ("Quantum Weird Patients, Not Particles!"), underscores the importance for both patients and medical professionals to remain aware of the condition's ever-changing nature.

Understanding this variability can prevent confusion when patients continue to experience dizziness even after successful treatments such as the Epley maneuver or an elimination diet. There are multiple examples and possibilities, but they all lead to the same response: continue with the vestibular migraine treatment regimen. Don't fall into the trap of thinking the condition has changed.

One of the biggest challenges for both patients and medical professionals is that there are no specific diagnostic tests, either physical examinations or laboratory tests, for vestibular migraine. As such, any diagnosis relies primarily on a patient's medical history and on ruling out other potential diagnoses. To address this challenge, I developed an algorithm to aid in diagnosing my patients. The initial version was crafted in 2004 and has since undergone several updates. The version presented below reflects the current iteration:

194 Dieterich M, Brandt T., Episodic vertigo related to migraine (90 cases): vestibular migraine? *J Neurol.* need full journal name here]. 246:883–892. DOI: 10.1007/s004150050478.

195 Neuhauser H., Leopold, M von Brevern, Arnold G., Lempert.T. (2001)The interrelations of migraine, vertigo, and migrainous vertigo. *Neurology.* 2001 Feb 27; 56(4):436-41. DOI: 10.1212/wnl.56.4.436.

Algorithm for Diagnosing Vestibular Migraine

Group A criteria

1. Dizziness

    a. Chronic, ongoing dizziness (4 wks to several yrs)

    b. Episodic episodes of dizziness (few sec to several days)

    c. Continuous dizziness after vertigo episodes (more than 1 day)

2. Vertigo

    a. Vertigo episodes of short duration (few sec to 15 min)

    b. Classical vestibular episode (15 min to 72 h)

    c. BPPV (Benign Paroxysmal Positional Vertigo)

Group B criteria

1. To fit at least one of the historical migraine definitions, according to the International Headache Society classification (lifetime diagnosis of migraine)

2. Presence of Migraine cohorts

    a. Migraine history in the first-degree relatives

    b. Presence of Motion sickness (including childhood)

Group C criteria

1. Ear symptoms without hearing loss

    a. Tinnitus or humming noise (uni- or bilateral, continuous or episodic)

    b. Pressure or fullness in ear (uni- or bilateral, continuous or episodic)

2. Ear symptoms with hearing loss

    a. Progressive sensorineural hearing loss

    b. Sudden sensorineural hearing loss

Wks (weeks), yrs (years), sec (seconds), min (minutes), h (hours), SBP (Systolic Blood Pressure,) DBP (Diastolic Blood Pressure)

I considered a patient to be experiencing vestibular migraine if they exhibited one of the criteria from group A plus the first criterion from group B, or one of the two criteria from group B-2 (Presence of Migraine cohorts) after other potential causes of vertigo/dizziness had been ruled out. They might exhibit one or more criteria from group C, or even none. Remember, vestibular migraine patients may show up only with ear symptoms without dizziness or vertigo from time to time.

An Algorithm? Et Tu, Alev?

Earlier in this book, I voiced criticism regarding existing diagnostic algorithms, prompting some readers to question my decision to create one of my own. However, in the realm of science, effective communication often necessitates speaking the language of science itself. Developing an algorithm provides a structured framework for conveying diagnostic processes, ensuring clarity and consistency in clinical practice. My algorithm, while straightforward, emphasizes the importance of excluding alternative causes of vertigo/dizziness, such as neurological conditions or surgical interventions, before considering a diagnosis of vestibular migraine (VM) and initiating appropriate treatment.

So, there has been some progress over the past decades in terms of formulating diagnostic criteria for vestibular migraine, but because they require classic migrainous headaches, it is still not enough. I know from the thousands of patients I have worked with since the beginning of my career and my personal experience that a "migraine headache" is not a prerequisite for a vestibular migraine diagnosis. Fortunately, if you check the recent literature, you will see that many clinics are modifying the diagnostic criteria in order to increase their ability to reduce the likelihood of VM patients being misdiagnosed or undiagnosed.[196]

In an article published in 2019, the University of Texas researcher Shin Beh wrote, "Either headache or vertigo of VM might present as the initial symptom, which did not occur in a fixed pattern. For most patients, the headache occurs several years before vertigo, while for some other patients, headache and vertigo always present simultaneously. A few of the patients might have vertigo earlier than the headache, and very rarely, patients might have recurrent vertigo or dizziness without headache. VM without aura are more common."[197] Shin Beh's highlighting of the variability in presentation among VM patients challenges traditional beliefs, suggesting that the onset of symptoms may not follow a fixed pattern. Some patients experience vertigo before or independent of headache episodes, contrary to conventional narratives. This nuanced understanding underscores the necessity for updated diagnostic criteria that accommodate the heterogeneity of VM presentations. While I may disagree with assertions like the rarity of recurrent vertigo without headache, the evolving discourse surrounding VM diagnosis signifies a significant step forward from previous consensus criteria established by organizations like the International Headache Society and Barany Society. By embracing a dynamic approach to diagnostics and remaining receptive to new evidence and insights, clinicians can enhance their ability to accurately identify and manage vestibular migraine, ultimately improving patient outcomes and quality of life.

196 Furman, J. M., Balaban, C. D. (2015). Vestibular migraine. *Annals of the New York Academy of Sciences*, 1343(1). DOI: 10.1111/nyas.12645.

197 Beh, S. C., (2019). Vestibular Migraine: How to Sort it Out and What to Do About it. *Journal of Neuro-ophthalmology*, 39(2). DOI: 10.1097/WNO.0000000000000791.

The Three Musketeers: Vertigo, Psychology, and Gender Bias

Psychology has long played a crucial role in understanding overall well-being throughout modern medical history. However, little attention has been given to psychological factors when addressing conditions such as vestibular migraine (VM). This oversight is noteworthy because patients experiencing relapsing or chronic vertigo and dizziness often concurrently suffer from anxiety and depression. Studies indicate a direct connection between the vestibular nuclei and the limbic system via the brainstem. For instance, Carey Balaban[198] of the University of Pittsburgh demonstrated in 2003 that stimuli affecting balance control could significantly influence ascending pathways associated with anxiety. It's imperative to recognize the profound stress of living with this condition, as it can markedly impact a patient's quality of life across multiple domains.

From both personal and professional encounters, I've observed that the emotional toll of "not being understood" or worse, "not being believed" by family and close friends can often outweigh the physical effects of the condition itself. Vertigo and dizziness are inherently subjective symptoms; while people can readily relate to pain, understanding the sensations of vertigo and dizziness, especially for those who have never experienced them, can be challenging. Even individuals who have encountered occasional vertigo/dizziness episodes may struggle to empathize with those experiencing chronic manifestations.

My personal and professional experience also tells me that women are particularly susceptible to encountering skepticism around their condition. This area has not been researched in sufficient depth to allow me to impress you with robust data, but my experience has been consistent enough that I have seen strong patterns emerge—and let's be honest, history is bursting at the seams with examples of women being on the receiving end of bias.[199]

---

198 Balaban, C. D. (2003). Neural substrates linking balance control and anxiety. January 2003 Physiology & Behavior, 77(4-5):469-75. https://doi.org/10.1016/s0031-9384(02)00935-6

199 https://theconversation.com/gender-bias-in-medicine-and-medical-research-is-still-putting-womens-health-at-risk-156495

However—and perhaps fortunately—the research we do have suggests that women are less likely than men to experience anxiety around their condition. In 2012, for example, the Swiss researcher Annette Kurre's research team published an article based on a study to examine gender differences in 202 patients with dizziness and unsteadiness regarding self-perceived disability, anxiety, and depression. The article states, "Both genders did not differ significantly in the mean level of self-perceived disability, anxiety, depression, and symptom severity. There was a tendency of a higher prevalence of abnormal anxiety and depression in men (23.7%; 28.9%) compared to women (14.5%; 15.3%). In men, the odd ratios (OR) was 8.2 (2.35–28.4). In women, chi-square statistics were not significant. The ORs (95% confidence intervals, CI, of abnormal anxiety and severe disability were 4.2 (1.9–8.9) in the whole sample, 8.7 (2.5–30.3) in men, and not significant in women." [200] In short, men are more inclined to abnormal anxiety and severe disability than women are, as Kurre's research showed us. (If statistics aren't your thing: An odds ratio (OR) is a measure of association between an exposure and an outcome. The OR represents the odds that an outcome will occur given a particular exposure, compared to the odds of the outcome occurring in the absence of that exposure. The confidence interval (CI) represents the accuracy or precision of an estimate.)

The psychological impact extends beyond emotional and mental health. It can also affect balance and motor control strategies in people with vestibular problems. Fear of falling (FOF) can make patients reluctant to move, which delays their spontaneous recovery (motor compensation) and hinders their ability to manage their daily activities.[201] Patients who worry about losing their balance or falling tend to develop protective behaviors that can lead to their changing their routines or habits, or even abandoning previously cherished activities. Many people with vestibular challenges

---

200 Kurre, A., Straumann, D., van Gool, C. J. A. W. (2012) Gender differences in patients with dizziness and unsteadiness regarding self-perceived disability, anxiety, depression, and its associations, *BMC Ear, Nose and Throat Disorders*. 12, 2. https://doi.org/10.1186/1472-6815-12-2.

201 Cheng, Y. Y., Kuo, C. H., Hsieh, W. L., Lee, S. D., Lee, W. J. (2012). Anxiety, depression, and quality of life (QoL) in patients with chronic dizziness. *Archives of Gerontology*. Elsevier. https://doi.org/10.1016/j.archger.2011.04.007.

are afraid to go outside alone. Or they may avoid going to certain places. Supermarkets, malls, and crowded open areas like bazaars or parking lots are particularly challenging areas because they can lead to sensory overload thanks to the sheer number of moving subjects (people, vehicles, etc.), not to mention noise and uneven surfaces. All these factors can have a negative impact on quality of life and, in the worst cases, lead to depression.[202]

One of the few points of consensus around VM in the medical community is that vertigo/dizziness can trigger or aggravate psychiatric problems and that they might not be correlated with the severity of a patient's symptoms. Jörg Wiltink of the Johannes Gutenberg-Universität Mainz conducted a large population-based study in 2009. He discovered that more than a quarter (28%) of dizziness patients reported that they had symptoms of an anxiety disorder and had increased healthcare use. Moreover, his research revealed that 18% of dizziness sufferers had panic disorder, 13% had a generalized anxiety disorder, and 9% had social anxiety.[203] These numbers are higher than in the normal (that is, healthy) population, but it is hard to say which problem develops first. We know that stress can trigger health problems, but health problems can make us anxious and stressed.

Beyond their impact on patients' general quality of life, these chronic conditions also impose serious economic burdens on patients, and as I'm sure you can imagine, that does nothing to improve their emotional and mental well-being.

The Old Gentleman in an Old Suit

I can still vividly recall the sight of his suit. It emitted a distinct aroma—a blend of Turkish coffee, tobacco, and the faint scent of old fabric—that instantly transported me back to my childhood. It was the kind of suit that

---

202 Cheng et al. (2012).

203 Wiltink, J., Tschan, R., Michal., M. (2009). Dizziness: anxiety, health care utilization, and health behavior--results from a representative German community survey. *Journal of Psychosomatic Research*. 66; pp. 417-424. https://doi.org/10.1016/j.jpsychores.2008.09.012.

seemed reserved for special occasions, tucked away in a closet and waiting patiently for its moment to shine. Despite its once-snug fit, it now hung loosely on his frame, a testament to the passage of time. This image stirred memories of my parents' emergency attire, kept for unforeseen events.

He was a refined gentleman in his early seventies, walking gracefully and carefully. His daughter and son-in-law accompanied him. He had been experiencing severe vertigo episodes with nausea, vomiting, and buzzing with hearing loss in his left ear for more than six months. When his symptoms first appeared, he and his family began to look for help for him. They had visited one of the university hospitals in Istanbul and some private neurology and OHNS practices, and he had undergone almost all the requisite diagnostic tests, plus a selection of others. His cranial MRI revealed very serious—in fact, alarming—shrinking of his brain tissue. All the physicians attributed his vertigo episodes to that finding. However, all his neurologic and cognitive functions were normal, and he did not report any episodes of amnesia. A retired accountant, he was living life as he always did, including helping his daughters file their taxes.

We began to talk about his medical history. He told me he had sporadic severe headaches in his forties and fifties and a similar period of vertigo episodes thirty years before.

"I was in Ankara at that time, and I went to Hacettepe University Hospital. They told me I had Meniere's disease, gave me some treatment, and I was completely healthy one month later. Even the ear buzzing stopped, and my hearing turned to normal."

I asked if the episodes had ever recurred in the three decades since. With absolute certainty he responded, "Never. Not once!"

I found that very interesting, and I asked whether he had been under stress at the time of his original vertigo episodes.

"Oh absolutely," he said. "I was working at the bank at that time, and our manager was a very difficult man. He made our lives hell for months, then the senior managers sent him away."

"Ok then, tell me what's been happening in your life in the last six months," I said.

"Well," he said, "nothing important. It's all good really and I'm happy. However, our youngest is getting married. My wife and I are very happy about it, but it is a bit hard, you know. We have four kids, and this is the last one to get married, and my wife and I will be alone from now on."

I smiled and tried to comfort him. "I think we've found the cause of your episodes. I don't believe it's your brain. I suspect you probably have a kind of migraine called vestibular migraine. It's usually diagnosed as Meniere's. Your stress most likely triggered it, but you'll be fine in no time." I wrote him a prescription and transferred him to my assistant for guidance on his diet, sleep, exposure to stress, exercise, etc. He arrived for his follow-up appointment three weeks later with a broad smile on his face. I am convinced that his recovery was due not only to the medication but also to my reassurance that his condition was not life-threatening and that he would recover.

CHAPTER 9

EVERYTHING OLD IS NEW AGAIN

I'm trying to adapt—they say you have to adapt to vertigo.
– Jason Day

Now, you might be wondering, "If my vertigo, or the vertigo in some of my patients, could be Vestibular Migraine, what differences does it make? Why is it important?"

I want to emphasize the crucial role of "accurate" diagnosis in facilitating effective treatment. Despite not fully grasping the exact mechanisms behind migraines, humanity has collected over twenty centuries of hands-on experience in managing and treating individuals with migraine symptoms.

Identifying vestibular migraine allows us to apply the same principles to their treatment, potentially sparing individuals like Jason Day from having to adapt to vertigo.

Everything might seem smooth and straightforward at this point — diagnose accurately, apply the known remedies, and voila! Another individual on the path to happiness and health.

But here's the real kicker: Navigating the intricacies of human nature, possibly the most complex aspect of our solar system, adds layers of intrigue and challenge to the whole process.

Oliver Sacks' words, "Many patients consider their migraines to occur 'spontaneously' and without cause. Such a view leads to scientific absurdity, emotional fatalism, and therapeutic impotence. We must assume that all episodes of migraine have real and discoverable determinants, however difficult their elucidation may be,"[204] encapsulate the timeless wisdom of dealing with migraine patients. However, viewing migraines as spontaneous and without cause implies a lack of control, turning individuals into helpless victims. But acknowledging a cause or trigger allows control and protection.

Indeed, I can proceed to provide guidance on the right and wrong things to do for vestibular migraine, listing common triggers like dietary restrictions, but why rush? While I will cover these aspects eventually, let's take the opportunity to delve deeper. Feel free to skip my jibber-jabber and jump straight to that section, but I'll pose the question once more—why? You invested in this book, so let's savor every drop and meet Dr. Groddeck.

Who draws the conclusion that I mentally medicate a human who has broken his leg, is very true—but I adjust the fracture and dress the wound. And then—I give him a massage, make exercises with him, give a daily bath to the leg, with water of 45 centigrade for half an hour, and I take care, that he does neither gorge nor booze, and every now and then I ask him: Why did you break your leg, you yourself?
– George Groddeck

---

204 Oliver Sacks, *Migraine.*

Dr. Groddeck's paragraph may seem unconventional and challenging to interpret at first. The concepts of mind-body connections and holographic medicine might appear unempirical to unfamiliar eyes and ears. However, I encourage you to keep aside bias and continue reading Lazslo Antonio Avila's wise words,[205] "The no man's land between body and mind, that uncharted territory where medicine merges with the humanities, raises many problems. Questions about the relationship between the somatic and the psychic have arisen for centuries, at least since the time of Descartes. Despite recent advances in both medicine and psychology, many problems remain unresolved. There is a deep-felt need for more comprehensive models, which integrate both theoretical and clinical perspectives on what it means to be human."

Suppose I were to critique modern medicine despite its remarkable progress in nearly all fields at a rapid pace. In that case, it has overlooked one crucial aspect: the comprehensive management of the patient as a "whole human." Drew Leder[206] in 1992 expressed, "Patients are often treated in a depersonalized, even dehumanized, fashion within the modern healthcare system. Their suffering is not heard and responded to; their wishes are not incorporated fully into treatment decisions; their resources for self-healing are not called into play".

While sounding somewhat harsh, this statement sadly holds the truth. There may be various explanations and excuses to cover this, such as economics, bureaucratization, technology, and modern medical training. While these explanations have some logic, they shouldn't excuse us, as current physicians, from remembering that our patients are complete humans—with bodies, psyches/minds, pasts, life choices, beliefs, habits, families, friends, environments, and more—all influencing their health and healing.

As mentioned earlier, working in a tertiary clinic meant most of my patients had previous diagnoses. One diagnosis that particularly bothered me was "Psychogenic Vertigo/dizziness."

205 Avila L.A. Georg Groddeck: originality and exclusion. *History of Psychiatry*, 14:1; 83-101.
206 Drew Leder. *The Body in Medical Thought and Practice*. Springer, August 31, 1992.

The diagnosis of "Psychogenic Vertigo/dizziness" subtly and offensively suggests that the patient's complaints have no biological basis, implying that the symptoms are entirely fabricated in their mind. While I am not a psychiatrist, I am familiar with conversion disorders. What perplexes me is that all the patients with this diagnosis were referred by OHNS doctors or neurologists, not by psychiatrists.

I label this ostensibly "benign" diagnosis as menacing because once someone's disorder is tagged as "Psychogenic," those around them tend to dismiss their complaints, making it challenging for the patient to receive the support needed for healing. Moreover, this diagnosis often coexists with depression, especially in chronic vertigo/dizziness patients. Please don't judge me; I'm not suggesting that psychology has no role in disease or healing. On the contrary, I want to emphasize that the psychology and biology of a patient are deeply intertwined.

Taking it a step further, I would argue that diagnoses like chronic subjective dizziness, phobic postural vertigo, subjective imbalance, and space-motion phobia may potentially be undiagnosed vestibular migraines. These manifestations might go unnoticed with conventional examinations and get erroneously classified as purely psychological problems. I hope this clarifies my intention.

Foucault[207] quips that the "man as a machine" belief (which has roots in the 17th century) in his *Discipline and Punish*; The Great Book of Man a Machine[208] was written simultaneously on two registers; the anatomico-metaphysical register, of which Descartes wrote the first pages and which the physicians and philosophers continued, and the technico-political register, which was constituted by a whole set of regulations and by empirical and calculated methods relating to the army, the school, and the hospital, for controlling or correcting the operations of the body."

---

207 M. Foucault, *Discipline and Punishment*. Vintage Books (April 25, 1995) 1, p. 136.
208 *Man a Machine*, written by Julien Offray de La Mettrie and first published in 1747.

Considering the human body as a machine can offer practical insights when understanding its anatomical or chemical workings. If viewed as a machine, even one of immense intricacy, the practitioner focuses on identifying and repairing the part that malfunctions. In this approach, other elements or the overall well-being of the "'machine" may not be a primary concern; the practitioner operates akin to a mechanic.

As medicine advances, our ability to address minuscule parts of the body grows, leading to increased focus on specific areas. Today, an OHNS surgeon faces the choice of specialization, whether in ear surgery, head and neck procedures, or exclusive dedication to endoscopic sinus surgeries. In contrast, five decades ago, OHNS surgeons received comprehensive training in microscopic and endoscopic surgeries, catering to adult and pediatric cases. The current trend of specialization enhances expertise in a specific area, allowing for concentrated efforts to achieve perfection. However, it also introduces a potential downside—overspecialization may create a sense of distance between healthcare professionals and their patients.

If you perceive your dizzy patient solely as another inner ear problem, unraveling the triggering factors and formulating effective treatment principles becomes an intricate task.

While discussing patient management, isn't it the perfect time to revisit history and recall the insights of medico-philosophers? Your enthusiasm is contagious!

Forgotten Gem: Medico-Philosophy

"The doctor is treating, but nature is healing."

"Natural forces within us are the true healers of disease."

"If anyone wants good health, one must first ask if he is willing to let go of what is the cause of his illness. Only then is it possible to help him."

"Before you heal someone, ask him if he's willing to give up the things that make him sick."

"If you are not your own doctor, you are a fool."

"Because the self-healing powers are understood and well known by the holistic physician, he can also prevent illness."

"The function of protecting and developing health must rank even above that of restoring it when it is impaired."

While these aphorisms and quotations may seem like "new age" knowledge to you, they were actually addressed to Hippocrates two millennia ago.[209]

It's interesting how some ideas in medicine are circling back to their origins. This forgotten wisdom has occasionally resurfaced through courageous physicians, although they haven't always been embraced by their colleagues with open arms and hearts. One such courageous figure was Georg Walther Groddeck. Let me introduce you to Groddeck's pathway; but first, let's get to know him.

There are apparently two essentially different causes (of illness),
an inner one, causa interna, which the man contributes to himself,
and an outer one, causa externa, which springs from his environment.
And accepting this clear distinction, we have thrown ourselves with raging
force upon the external causes...And the causa interna, that we have
forgotten. Why? Because it is not pleasant to look within ourselves.
– G.W. Groddeck (1866–1934)

I encountered the quote by Groddeck many years ago in Oliver Sacks' *Migraine,* and that paragraph truly struck me. Now, I want you to explore the life of Dr. Georg Groddeck a bit. Despite his invaluable contributions, I believe he didn't receive his deserved appreciation. It's crucial to navigate the history of medicine and acknowledge the individuals who paved the

---

209 Ventegodt S., (2020)

way for discoveries and deep understanding. Their hard work has gradually enhanced the comfort and well-being of humanity, piece by piece. Respecting and remembering them is an ode to our medical heritage.

Lazslo Antonio Avila[210] wrote, "The German physician Georg Walther Groddeck was a polemical freethinker; nurtured in a rich intellectual atmosphere, he produced medical and literary texts of great originality and interest throughout his 68 years. His works, which interlinked and interacted with each other, sought understanding of the symbolic aspects of human life in both health and illness."

Groddeck,[211] born in Baden Baden, south Germany in 1866, was a physician, a pioneer of psychoanalysis and psychosomatic medicine, and a prolific writer. During medical school, his favorite teacher was Ernst Scheweninger, a renowned doctor who treated Otto Von Bismarck. Despite Scheweninger's reputation for being oppressive and harsh, he surprisingly embraced the medical motto "Nil Nocera" (not to harm). His treatments primarily involved diets, massages, and hydrotherapy. Avila aptly summarized Scheweninger's perspective: "Schweninger's view was that nature was the source of all healing... the patient possessed the means for the cure, leaving the doctor the task of discovering the barriers that impeded this natural process." During this era, medicine underwent a "scientific revolution" marked by continuous discoveries, advancements in various medical fields, and a focus on pathogenic agents. Schweninger's approach, deemed "natural medicine," was seen as a craft trade and considered "anti-scientific" amid the prevailing scientific trends.

Groddeck adored him and considered him as the "greatest living physician." Therefore, he adopted Scheweninger's rejection of orthodox medicine and embraced the naturopathic medicine approach, but he built his unique psychosomatic approach. In his sixtieth birthday celebration, Ernst Simmel said, "Groddeck may be permitted to style himself 'wild' in relation

210 Georg Groddeck: originality and exclusion. LA Avila, M Winston. *History of Psychiatry*, 2003. journals.sagepub.com.

211 Georg Groddeck, M Grotjahn, *Psychoanalytic Pioneers*. 1966 books.google.com.

to the movement of which he is a supporter—in the sense that he owes his training to no one but himself... which impels him to the action where others throw up a case as hopeless or disguise their real helplessness under the cover of "accurate diagnosis."

I want to share one of his patient's stories here for excitement, to stir the muddy waters, and leave the whole interpretation to you. "One of his patients, a woman, suffered from severe, generalized edema, despite treatment of her heart condition with medication and with the special massage Groddeck had learned from Scheweninger. The patient then confessed her 'sin' that she had vowed to remain a virgin and become a nun, but she had since married and was no longer a virgin. After her 'confession,' she passed enormous quantities of urine, a veritable 'sin fluid' was released. Within twenty-four hours, she had lost fifteen pounds."[212]

Well, it sounds too good to be true, but that was Dr. Groddeck, and he wrote it down. It is impossible to go back there and control whether this story is true, but I can infer that we still don't know our brains' capabilities. I believe he witnessed that woman's impressive healing process. You may like his work, or you can shrug your shoulders, but don't forget, he dedicated himself to "lost cases," chronically ill patients who came to him as their last resort. His deficiency may be his focusing only on the psychology of his patients; although this approach helped develop psychotherapeutic treatment, he may miss the patient's circumstances. Hard to say. I think his most practical conclusion, which one can brew onto his long career, even though it was not entirely an original one, but long forgotten and dismissed (and still so), was that diseases were always the expression of suffering in both body and soul and to be sick comprises the whole person and not some biological system alone.

Sadly, it has been nearly a hundred years since Dr. Groddeck, but integrative medicine is still in its "early" stage of development. You can find integrative clinics; they are primarily under the umbrella of academic institutions, but unfortunately, they are very limited in number.

---

212 Georg Groddeck: Originality and exclusion. LA Avila, M Winston, *History of Psychiatry*. 2003, journals.sagepub.com.

I hoped I could help him, which meant helping him to help himself
because, with mind-body disorders, a doctor cannot cure a patient.
It is the suffering patient who must come to understand his malady...
and by understanding it, banish it.
– John E. Sarno

I had a ringside seat to observe vertigo and dizziness for all these years, and I, myself, endured it too. I always tried to explain to my patients that they are the source and principal healers of their Vestibular Migraine episodes.

I had an ample numbers of patients to demonstrate to me that if you have a mutual understanding with your patient and if you can persuade them that they have control over this debilitating disorder, this is the exact moment your patient begins to heal.

But I'm Good!

Knowledge of the disorder was essential to successful treatment.
– John E. Sarno, MD

Mr. G.D. was in his mid-thirties, tall, handsome, refined, well-educated, and working in a high position in a demanding sector. He had a bitter divorce more than a year ago and has been dizzy since that time. He tried numerous physicians, and he had all kinds of diagnostic tests you could ever think of for a dizzy patient except examination with VNG; all were normal, and his diagnosis was written solid: "psychogenic dizziness." He doesn't have much hope that this dizziness will ever be gotten rid of, but he heard about me and wanted to try. He had an interesting family history with a mom who had migraine headaches and a couple of vertigo/dizziness episodes, diagnosed in a wide spectrum of syndromes from BPPV to vestibular neuritis; his big sister had one Meniere's episode (!) many years ago.

On the examination with VNG, he had an unchanging left-beating nystagmus in all positions.

Back in the interview room, I told him all about vestibular migraine and the triggers responsible for his year-long dizziness; he thanked me and left the office. A couple of weeks later, he came for the control examination. I spoke with him as usual before the examination. He was free from his dizziness; he was so happy and thankful and asking for the future direction. There was no nystagmus on the test. He should have abided by all the rules that we recommended. I began to check him by asking about the things he should have been doing since he left the office, AKA my "written commands":

How was your sleep? Did you regulate it?

Well, not exactly; I had an intercontinental business meeting, flew to the USA and stayed a week... But I'm good.

Ok, how was your diet? Could you adapt it?

Well, I genuinely tried, but you know there were business lunches and dinners, and it is nearly impossible to find something to eat with a rational level of salt when you have to eat out... But I'm good.

OMG, Ok, how about drinking then?

Well, I should admit that I drank only white wine; believe me, I'm good.

I did believe him; how couldn't I? He was free from nystagmus, ergo dizziness. He asked me what he should do from now on. I said, keep going; you are doing the exact right thing, whatever it is.

I didn't see him again, but he called me once a year for three years to inform me that he was still "good." He was one of my patients who taught me a lot and made me smile whenever I remember.

CHAPTER 10

FIGHTING BACK AGAINST VESTIBULAR MIGRAINE

*Being a physician involves much more than handing out diagnosis
and treatment; it involves playing a role in some of the most intimate
decisions of a patient's life. This requires a considerable amount of human
delicacy and judgment, no less than medical judgment and knowledge.*
– Oliver Sacks

Vertigo Episodes, Puzzle Boards, and the Anna Karenina Principle

I use the metaphor of a "puzzle board" to help my patients understand the formation of a vestibular migraine episode, and it has proven effective every time. This metaphor serves as the best way to create a mental image, allowing them to grasp how various factors combine to stage a vestibular migraine display.

If you are one of the vestibular migraine (VM) puzzle board carriers, you are likely born with that board, probably genetically transferred to you through your parents' DNA. Like all other puzzle games, this board can exhibit the full features of a VM episode picture, manifesting as any kind of peripheral vertigo episode, dizziness, or aural fullness with or without low-frequency hearing loss. All that is needed is the puzzle pieces to complete to create the full picture of a vertigo episode.

In the words of Leo Tolstoy's iconic opening sentence from *Anna Karenina*, "All happy families are alike; each unhappy family is unhappy in its own way." This sentiment is known as the Anna Karenina Principle. The Anna Karenina Principle suggests that successful outcomes result from avoiding numerous possible pitfalls. Taking marriage as the original example, these pitfalls can span various aspects of life such as economic stability, parenting strategies, religious or political beliefs, fidelity, and many more. Applied to vestibular migraine (VM), just one last puzzle piece (specific trigger) can start an episode, and results in Anna Karenina's unhappy family in its own way.

These puzzle pieces can be anything that affects stress hormone levels, ranging from stressful conditions in everyday life to over-fatigue, irregular eating, and sleeping patterns, working or living out of the circadian rhythm, or even simple seasonal changes. Usually, it takes time for the puzzle pieces to come together gradually, and the last piece could be a seemingly innocent factor, such as one glass of wine or a nice cheese board. When you tell your patient that their Thursday dinner triggered their episode, it may sound unbelievable because it wasn't the first time they ate or drank the same or similar things. However, when other factors have prepared the basis, one last drop can easily start the chain reaction of an episode.

As you can consider, some of these factors (genes, seasons, our boss) are out of our control. Still, fortunately, the remaining parts of these puzzle pieces are under our control, like arranging our sleep schedules, learning to cope with stress, and our trigger foods and drinks. Even at times, a specific type of food or drink could be the last piece of the puzzle to independently complete the picture (vertigo/dizziness episode) to trigger a vestibular episode.

I always aimed to convey to my patients that they are the source and healer of their disorder, a belief I genuinely hold. I successfully connected with the majority of my patients, and as they witnessed their ability to alter the course of their disease, the struggle against vertigo/dizziness found resolution. For patients, recognizing this mutual understanding and instilling confidence that they have control over this debilitating curse marks the precise starting point of the healing process.

Once Upon a Time, Food Was Medicine. Could It Still Be So?

Humans tried to heal themselves along with history like all other living organisms, but let's give us our due: we tried much more creative ways for sure. However, it may not be very exceptional, since most mammals are doing the same; food has always been the most popular. Yet, interestingly, many ancient recipes harbored mysterious wisdom. For example, there is an impressive historical story behind the treatment of night blindness with food that later enabled the discovery of vitamin A. The first written source about the remedy of night blindness is in the ancient Egyptian papyrus Kahun[213] (1825 BC), which refers to "instructions for a woman, cannot see, *to eat the raw liver* of a donkey." And in the famous Egyptian Papyrus, Ebers[214] (1500 BC) recommends, "Roasted ox liver, pressed, applied (topical to the eye)" for the night blindness.

Later, in the Middle Ages, the Dutch Physician Jacob van Maerlandt (1235–1299)[215] wrote the following poem recommending eating liver:

Who does not at night see right

Eats the liver of the goat

He will then see better at night.

---

213 Nunn JF. Ancient Egyptian Medicine. Landon: British Museum Press; 1996. In press.

214 Ebell B. *The Greatest Egyptian Medical Document*. Copenhagen: Munksgaard and Oxford University Press; 1937. The Papyrus Ebers.

215 Lindeboom CA. Historical milestones in the treatment of night blindness. *Clin Med.* 1984;19:40–9.

In the late 19th and early 20th centuries, extensive research efforts led to the discovery of vitamin A. Its deficiency was identified as the cause of night blindness, a condition effectively treated with vitamin A supplementation. Vitamin A exists in two main forms: provitamin A carotenoids (found in vegetables like carrots), and preformed vitamin A. Preformed Vitamin A (including retinol and retinoic acid) is the most active form of Vitamin A, primarily present in animal-based foods, particularly in the liver. The liver, rich in Vitamin A, stores approximately 50–85% of body retinol.[216]

This remarkable historical narrative emphasize the importance of exploring the archives of medicine. A similar exploration could shed light on the understanding and treatment of migraines, including vestibular migraines.

As mentioned, at least four well-known medical papyri mention migraine (hemi-cranial) headaches:[217] Ebers, Beatty, Leiden, and Deir el-Medina. Although other migraine symptoms were not indicated in these papyri, in Ebers, papyri "spitting mouth" was written twice with the headache and probably referring to vomiting.

When it comes to treatment, although there is a list of animal and plant remedies for the treatment of headaches listed in Ebers, we don't know whether Egyptian doctors were using them by ingestion. There is a famous paragraph in the Ebers papyrus describing a remedy for one side of the head: "Skulls of catfish; were heated until they turned to ashes and boiled with oil; the head is rubbed therewith for four days," so we can infer that all mentioned remedies were applied directly to the patient's head.

Indeed, no written evidence shows us the Egyptians had the same insight for migraine in treating night blindness; although they were using "food," they were doing that externally.

Let's explore ancient Greeks, starting with the father of physicians, Hippocrates. "Let food be thy medicine, and medicine be thy food," is a

---

216 H.A. Hajar Al Binali, M.D. Night Blindness and Ancient Remedy. *Heart Views*. 2014 Oct-Dec; 15(4): 136–139.

217 Karenberg, A., Leitz, C., Headache in magical and medical papyri of Ancient Egypt *Cephalalgia*. 11/2001, Volume 21, Issue 9.

well-known pearl of wisdom attributed to him.[218] However, some scholars argue whether Hippocrates said that or not; this aphorism undoubtedly formed the basis of ancient Greek/Hippocratic medicine.[219]

In 2005, Alain Touwaide[220] wrote the assay known as "Regimen," revealing the analysis and role of what we now call nutraceuticals (superfoods). This discovery is believed to trace back to the late fifth or the early fourth century BCE. Similarly, in his review of the science of folic acid, Mark Lucock[221] highlighted that around 2500 years ago, Hippocrates first espoused the philosophy of "food as medicine," which fell into obscurity by the 19th century. The initial half of the 20th century witnessed the discovery of essential elements and vitamins, especially in the context of deficiency diseases. Lucock concludes his discussion by quoting Hippocrates: "Let food be thy medicine and medicine be thy food."

In the same issue of the *British Medical Journal*, editor Richard Smith[222] put it wisely, "Although many patients are convinced of the importance of food in both causing and relieving their problems, many doctors' knowledge of nutrition is rudimentary. Most feel much more comfortable with drugs than foods, and the "food as medicine" philosophy of Hippocrates has been largely neglected." But fortunately, this "neglect" has begun to reverse in recent decades.

During the Hippocratic era, two medical schools, Cos and Cnidus, coexisted, both subscribing to the "four humors" theory established by Empedocles (c. 490–430 BC). However, the Cnidians were empiricists— observers and classifiers. Hippocrates, affiliated with the Coan school,

218 Jones WHS. *Hippocrates*. Vol. I–IV. London: William Heinemann, 1923-1931.

219 Ventegodt S. Comparison of the medical principles of the ancient Egyptian and the ancient Greek medicine based on the medical papyri. *Journal of alternative medicine research*. 04/2020, Volume 12, Issue 2.

220 Touwaide A.,Appetiti E., Food and medicines in the Mediterranean tradition. A systematic analysis of the earliest extant body of textual evidence. *Journal of Ethnopharmacology*. 06/2015, Volume 167.

221 Lucock M., Science, medicine, and the future. Is folic acid the ultimate functional food component for disease prevention? *BMJ*. 2004 Jan 24; 328(7433): 211–214.

222 Richard S., Let food be thy medicine. *BMJ*, 01/2004, Volume 328, Issue 7433.

dedicated himself to studying the causes of diseases through direct observation and inference.[223]

While Hippocrates[224] was the first to use the term "Migraine" and describe most migraine headache symptoms, including visual disturbances now known as aura, Aretaeus of Cappadocia emerged as a superstar in the history of migraines.[225]

Approximately two-hundred years later, Aretaeus reviewed the treatment of migraines in the "Manual for the Treatment of Chronic Diseases," Book A. He begins with the importance of the head. "The more necessary the head is to life, the more agonizing it may be as a result of the disease. In the beginning, the patient experiences little trouble from diseases that originate in the head, a little pain, buzzing in the ears and a heavy feeling." He continues, discussing surgery, detailing bleeding sites and techniques, some of which are rather grim. However, my primary focus in that chapter was on the "diet," and I discovered more than I had anticipated.

He begins the nutrition section with wine, stating, "First, have the patient drink wine for two days," and then he recommends, "Then, order the patient to eat more for three or four days." Following this, he suggests emptying the gastrointestinal system, saying, "Subsequently, have him empty the hiera* with melikraton.* For this medicine, in particular, removes the nourishment of the disease from the head." Well, it seems that two millennia ago, at least the first six days of treatment looked festive, doesn't it? The following purgation ruins the fun, but the previous six days shouldn't be so bad.

*(Hiera, the "sacred" purgative, consisted of aloe and some aromatic substances. *Melikraton, or hydromel, is a mixture of honey and water.)

---

223 Food and medicines in the Mediterranean tradition. A systematic analysis of the earliest extant body of...by Touwaide, Alain; Appetiti, Emanuela. *Journal of ethnopharmacology.* 06/2015, Volume 167.

224 Allory AL., Hippocrates, *Concerning Migraine.* Thesis, Paris, 1859.

225 Koehler P.J., van de Wiel T.W.M., 2001

While my initial intention was to explore diets, the progression of treatment after applying the medicines is too intriguing not to share. Be honest, if you learn something like this, wouldn't you want to share it with your readers? Aretaeus continues to outline his treatment regime, "When the patients have gradually recovered a little, let them engage in exercises for the chest and shoulders while standing, move their hands, do dumbbell exercises, jump, and turn the body at the same time according to the instructions. Massage the thighs at the beginning and the end and the head halfway through the exercises. Oil their heads with pitch frequently. Also, make the head red, one time by rubbing it in with mustard, adding the double quantity of bread so that he can bear the heat, the other time by smearing medicines like the compound that consists of wolf's milk, and pellitory. The juice of thapsia eases the pain that occasionally appears and also episodes the disease at its root. This also occurs with all medicines that have been made with it, and that swell the skin and cause skin eruption resembling acne." See? After six fun days of eating and drinking, if you still have headache, things get nasty. I'm sure his patients had been happy and would accept all the diets I suggest later to you instead of this lovely regimen. (Yup, I'm leading up to my way.)

Now, let's explore the diet. Aretaeus wrote, "The diet has to be scanty in each type of pain. The patient should drink little, only water, especially some time before taking some drug. They have to abstain from anything acrid: onions, garlic, and juice of silphium.* They do not have to abstain from mustard entirely. For the acrimony of mustard is not only good for the stomach, but also it is not unpleasant for the head, as it liquefies and promotes the evaporation or excretion through the intestine of phlegm." I would like to highlight something here; it looks like Aretaeus, or maybe all physicians of his time, were trying to secrete/excrete some fluid from the patient's body; probably they were aware of the role of fluid retention in migraine episodes.

(*Silphium was a plant used in classical antiquity as a seasoning, perfume, aphrodisiac, and medicine.)

Continuing with Aretaeus, who wrote, "Among pulses, beans are the worst; subsequently, lentils, although they have some favorable characteristics with respect to digestion and secretion, bring about the fullness of the head and headache. If lentils are cooked with pepper, they don't need to be omitted from the diet." As you can see, he once again emphasizes the elimination of excess bodily fluids. He continued with food suggestions: "Agreeable food includes bearded wheat, washed and with as much wine and honey as will taste well to the patients. Bearded wheat as porridge, and bearded wheat with simple sauces are agreeable as well. Spices that are found in karykeia* are also good: caraway, coriander, aniseed, and celery. Even better than these are mint and pennyroyal with their nice scent; they contain something that promotes micturition and flatulence."

(*A dish in which the karuke is used; a sauce invented by the Lydians, also called a Lydian sauce, composed of blood and spices.)

I'll gracefully sidestep the topic of flatulence for now—its importance is yet to be unraveled. But let's focus on the fascinating emphasis on micturition (urination). Water and salt balance has pivotal importance in conditions like epilepsy, migraine, hypertension, and the enigmatic "Meniere's disease." Hence his choice of foods promoting urination is fascinating and impressive. If you remember the "Meniere's Disease, water, salt, and a Little Bit of Insight" in Chapter 5, starting in the 1940s, restricting salt intake—the Furstenberg regimen—emerged as the cornerstone of Meniere's treatment and continues to hold its fundamental role. This regimen serves as the first aid for Meniere's patients, aiming to control water retention.

The intriguing historical query lingers: Did Furstenberg draw inspiration from Aretaeus? While the answer remains elusive, the shared goal is evident—to restrict or prevent water retention.

Let's dig deeper into Aretaeus; the following paragraphs unveil even more intriguing insights. He begins with a timeless caution, "Meat that causes trouble includes all the meat that has been preserved too long." I'll exemplify contemporary diet suggestions later, but the exclusion of preserved meats (probably contain ample amounts of salt) is undeniably intriguing, don't you think?

His gastronomic guidance persists, urging, "Give fresh meat. Cocks. Among birds, wood pigeons, common pigeons, and all sorts, as long as they are not too fat." Aretaeus suggests poultry, much like me, but It seems he either never encountered a "chicken a la regret" patient (page 179), or intriguingly, he did and opted for cocks over chickens! Aretaeus seems to know something we're still in the dark about!

The mystery deepens as Aretaeus asserts, "Milk and cheese cause headaches." While I, a lactose-intolerant myself, steer clear of milk, the condemnation of cheese, a notorious migraine trigger since his time, is noteworthy.

Aretaeus extends his culinary counsel to fish and veggies, recommending "rock fishes" (likely Mediterranean species) and all cooked veggies that promote, guess what? Yes, "micturition and defecation." Among raw vegetables, lettuce reigns supreme, while roots—radish, rapeseed, and carrots—are condemned for promoting micturition but inducing a feeling of fullness. Aretaeus' dietary wisdom, resonating across centuries, unveils a nuanced understanding of the intricate relationship between food and well-being.

We are well aware that wines, especially red wines, are triggers for migraine headaches (including vestibular migraines). Surprisingly, Aretaeus seems to have known this too, as he wrote, "Among the wines, white wine that is thin, sweet, and a little astringent is permitted so that the intestines do not become obstructed." While I can't comment on "obstructed intestines," I'm optimistic about white wines (I experimented personally; I need a smiley emoticon here!). Joking aside, my experience with patients aligns with this: white wine is often a safer alternative, especially if consumed with ice. Romans adopted a similar practice to elongate dinners without risking getting drunk (wise people!). However, as you'll discover later, with self-awareness, you might find intervals when you can safely enjoy a glass of merlot or cabernet (or whatever you like).

I must admit, Aretaeus perspective on desserts surprised me a bit; "All desserts, except all kinds of dates, cause headaches. Figs and grapes in fall are beneficial, and all that is best in only one season." While excessive carbohydrate intake is generally not recommended for anyone, migraineur or not, it's intriguing to consider why dates are exempted (perhaps due to their higher glycemic incidence or some ancient wisdom). And Aretaeus' final say, "Exuberance is bad whatever one eats, even if it is healthy food. Even worse is when the food is badly digested." As you see, he didn't fail us on his last remark, either. I have no idea what he tried to point out with the "badly digesting," but whatever, I have great respect for this guy.

About a hundred years after Aretaeus, Galen was born nearly in the same land: Pergamon, Anatolia. He was a physician, surgeon, and philosopher and is regarded as one of the most accomplished and prolific researchers and medical writers of his time.

Before delving into his essays, I must shed light on his personality a bit, as he was likely one of the most meticulous, detail-oriented, and perfectionist writers you'll ever encounter.

Julius Rocca [226] wrote a review essay on Mark Grant's "Galen on Food and Diet" in 2003. His essay begins by highlighting Galen's perfectionism: "One would not expect a reference to Aristophanes' "Merchant Ships" in a discussion on the properties of wild chickling (arakos), unless, that is, the writer in question is Galen."

This reference, as Rocca points out, is found in Book I of Galen's "On the Powers of Foodstuffs (De alimentis facultatibus)." Galen wrote, "I have found the last syllable of the word arakos written with k in the "Merchant Ships" by Aristophanes where it reads: 'wild chikling, wheat, pearl barley, groats, one-seeded wheat, darnel, and fine flour.' The seed is similar to that of a chickling, and some people do not think they are separate species, for the general use and power of wild chickling is similar to that of a chickling,

---

226 Julius Rocca. *Early Science, and Medicine, Galenic Dietetics. BRILL.* Online Publication Date: 01 Jan 2003. Volume 8: Issue 1, Article Type: Research Article, Pages: 44–51.

except that wild chickling is harder and more difficult to boil, and so is harder to digest than chickling."

Rocca interprets this as "This arguably tells us more about Galen than about wild chickling, for it illustrates not only Galen's desire to cite a literary source, reinforcing his image as an erudite physician but his obsessive, Galenic, attention to detail, which reinforces his image of near omniscience." Nothing better can be said.[227],[228]

Galen authored three books on the "Power of Food," which offer valuable insights into the principles of medicine in the second-century Roman Empire. During Galen's time, dietetics served not only as an adjunct to medical treatment, as they do today, but as a treatment modality in themselves. However, a constant in the history of medicine is physicians' dissatisfaction with their peers' works, and—of course—Galen was no exception. In Book 1, he criticized, "A considerable number of the most outstanding physicians have written about the powers of foods. Yet they have set down their ideas in a great deal of haste, even though this is probably the most important of all medical subjects." His discontent and complaint echo through the centuries in these words.[229]

While Hippocrates, Galen, and many others contributed thousands of pages on the relationship between food and health, Mark Grant notes, "Many historians concede that palliative care by Galen would have been far preferable to anything that was to be available until the closing years of the nineteenth century."

227 *Galen: Powell., O., ,On the Properties of Foodstuffs* Cambridge University Press 2003

228 Grant M., *Galen on Food and Diet.* London: 214 pp., bibl., index. New York/London: Routledge, 2000.

229 Scarborough J., On the Properties of Foodstuffs ("De alimentorum facultatibus") (review). *Bulletin of the History of Medicine. Johns* Hopkins University Press. Volume 79, Number 2, Summer 2005.

Alev Uneri

Of Course There Were Surgeons: The More The Merrier!

I said that humans were much more creative to treat and heal themselves than other mammals at the beginning of this chapter, even their close cousins. One of the "creative" ways is undoubtedly the surgery. It is hard to say when and how surgery became an option for humans, but it has probably been used since the dawn of civilization. It is easier to understand to try to operate the wounds—possibly it was created out of necessity—but it is hard to understand trying to operate on everything, let me be honest, usually without a clue. Consider the early surgical interventions for Meniere's disease shortly after its identification. These efforts reflect the impatience and genius inherent in human nature. The quest for shortcuts that align with evolutionary plans to achieve maximum gain with minimal effort is a characteristic feature.

Imagine discovering a shortcut to eliminate debilitating migraines—a quick solution that bypasses the need to memorize extensive food options, eliminate favorite foods, meticulously prepare recipes, and wait for results. The inclination to explore such shortcuts might explain the historical attempts at surgical interventions, even in Aretaeus' time. Humans, driven by curiosity and a desire for efficient solutions, have always sought innovative paths to address health challenges.

Although surgery has no role in the contemporary treatment of migraines (vestibular migraines), delving into Aretaeus' era and its surgical approaches offers a curious journey into the past. However, be prepared for some savagery that might make you grateful not to have lived in that time. Here's a glimpse: "Consequently, you have to shave off the hair (which yet on its own is good for the head) and cauterize superficially down to the muscles. If you wish to cauterize down to the bone, carry it out at a site where there are no muscles. For if you burn muscles, you will provoke cramps. When you have cauterized superficially, subsequently pour much odoriferous white wine with rose oil on the spot. You have to wet a small linen cloth, lay it on the burns and leave it for two days. If there are deep burns, scatter salt on leaves of leek and pulverize them, grease a small linen cloth with it, and lay it on the burns. Apply wax of rose oil on the superficial burns and lentils with honey on the deep burns two days later." Quite an eye-opener, isn't it?

For the sake of curiousness, here is another: "The meal has to be simple, although wine should go with it to stimulate the stomach, as this also suffers. If, in the meantime, the patient has regained strength, administer the usual laxative, scatter a lot of soda in it, or pour two drops of melted resin of turpentine. The subsequent day, to bleed the nose, push the instrument, a long stiletto inside. If one does not carry these, take the shaft of a thick goose feather, scrape off a bit from the outer layer, and make notches that result in teeth like on a saw. Subsequently, push the shaft inside the nose up to the ethmoid bones (OMG!!!!) and move it with both hands to create scratches at that site. In this way, a lot of blood will be discharged quickly, as many small veins end there, and the site is soft and easy to injure. Laymen, too, have many ways to injure their noses. They do it with raw plants and desiccated bay leaves, which they push inside with their hands and then move vigorously. When you have drawn the required amount of blood (you have to draw half a cotula [16.5 cubic inches], rub in the nose with a sponge with oxycraton, or blow a kind of dry styptic remedy inside, gall-apple, a piece of alum, or blossom of the wild pomegranate." Quite a unique historical approach!

Surgery for migraine headaches must be as old as the headache itself, but evidently it was a well-accepted and extensively used treatment around 200 AD, as you can read from Aretaeus: "The remedies you have to lay on a scar will be described elsewhere. Some physicians incise down to the bone on the forehead along the border of the hair. They abrade or chisel the bone down to the diploe and let flesh grow over the place. Others perforate the bone down to the meninges. (OMG! again.) These are hazardous treatments." (Of course! Aretaeus, obviously!) "You have to apply them when the headache persists after all that has been done; the patient keeps courage, and the body is vigorous." Now you know and possibly are grateful for modern medicine.

Your Plate and Your Vertigo: Is There a Connection?

Let's fly seventeen-hundred years forward from our Aretaeus to the other legendary guy of migraine, Oliver Sacks; in *Migraine*, he has a chapter about migrainous foods, which you can apply one-to-one to vestibular migraine without question.

He candidly wrote, "Experience since the first edition of this book has made clear that there can be specific food reactions and that these may have a clearly defined chemical mechanism. The phrase 'Chinese restaurant syndrome' has become very familiar (though very distressing to Chinese restaurants!). Many persons, and an especially high proportion of migraineurs, may show severe reactions to Chinese meals. In milder cases, there is just a feeling of malaise, with some shivering, pallor, borborygmus, and nausea; in more severe cases, there may be absolute prostration, with severe visceral and vascular upset (including a typical candidly faintness, if not actual 'fainting.' It is clear that such reactions come in the 'borderlands' of migraine and resemble the 'migranoid reactions,' the vasovagal episodes, the nitritoid crises, and so on …. It is evident that one is seeing a parasympathetic or 'vagotonic' response—and one to which migraineurs are especially prone." Does it sound familiar to you?

The term "Chinese Restaurant Syndrome" is now outdated; it's more commonly known as the monosodium glutamate (MSG) symptom complex. Thus, we understand that not every Chinese meal will lead to this syndrome. Despite its unnatural nature, MSG is not a toxic ingredient. It is, let's say, unnatural, like many millions of other food additives. Additionally, MSG is a handy flavor enhancer and a staple in South Asian cuisine, with most people tolerating it perfectly well. However, if you have vestibular migraines, you should be cautious with MSG, especially during vulnerable phases like stressful periods, seasonal transitions, or when experiencing sleeping and eating irregularities.

MSG is not the sole concern regarding food and migraines. Starting with Aretaeus, individuals, particularly physicians, interested in migraines wrote about the power of foods that make patients sick. We certainly know that some foods are common migraine triggers, such as aged cheese. In the 1950s, cheese and some other foods were deemed dangerous for patients receiving monoamine oxidase inhibitor (MAOI) antidepressants due to the risk of provoking a sudden and dangerous rise in blood pressure. Although these drugs (MOAIs) were extraordinarily effective, they were eventually abandoned and replaced with much safer but less potent tricyclic antidepressants.

It's essential to note that not all migraine sufferers, but only some of them and only at specific times, exhibit MSG intolerance, cheese intolerance, or other food sensitivities. Food sensitivities may be influenced by digestion, gut physiology, gut microbiome, and brain chemistry, making it challenging to pinpoint the type of reaction and when it occurs.

The Fishy Tale of Vertigo on a Plate

I'll call her our big sister, Flowery, because she is our family's caring and loving big sister, without blood relation (sometimes it is better, right?). I have known her for over 35 years, which I praise daily. I know her closely, and I have never seen a migraine headache episode from her. Still, she has two sisters (blood relative siblings), one younger and one older, and both had terrible migraine headaches in all these years.

After menopause, Flowery began to have vertigo episodes, not often, but nasty ones with nausea and vomiting. We even had to put her on IV (intravenous 5% dextrose) a few times due to excessive vomiting. It was relentless, at least a whole day. After one or two episodes, we found the trigger, which happened to be a specific kind of fish (unfortunately, which is very, very delicious). Still, this particular species was triggering her episodes. After I realized that, I updated my diet handouts as you expect and put (certain kinds of) fish in the "don't" part.

I should add a particular memory from my childhood: my auntie (who had migraine headaches and later vertigo) was afraid to eat fish whenever she cooked it. She had that scare; if you eat fish with dairy (milk or yogurt especially), it may cause horrible food poisoning, which she described as vertigo, nausea, and vomiting. Probably, she had an episode with a fish meal like our Flowery in the past, and that fear stayed with her.

Later, while I was working with vertigo patients, I saw many patients who had had unique "food poisonings!" in their past and never knew that they had vestibular migraine episodes (along with their physicians, obviously). I call these alleged food poisonings unique because my patients were the only ones poisoned (!) with the same meal while others devoured heartily.

While addressing triggering foods, I should tell you one more story.

The Fowl Play: Chicken à La Regret

It must have been the early 2000s; I was at the institute, trying to advise my vestibular migraine (VM) patient on what he should do in the upcoming weeks before his follow-up appointment. As I went through the instructions outlined in the pamphlet prepared for VM patients, including a list of foods to avoid, the patient interrupted me with a familiar question: "OMG! What am I going to eat!!??"

Patient interaction, no matter how routine, always holds surprises. This time was no different. As I confidently listed permissible foods, emphasizing the abundance of chicken, the patient interjected, "Oh, no! I can't eat chicken. Every time I eat it, I vomit."

I knew the toll that prolonged vertigo could take on patients—how it could breed feelings of depression, anxiety, and helplessness. Glancing at my assistant, we shared a knowing look; encountering such "interesting" patients had become a part of our daily routine. I didn't push the issue further, but inwardly, I couldn't help but doubt the sincerity of the patient's claim.

Fast forward several years, perhaps three or four. I examined a new patient in her late thirties, accompanied by her mother and daughter. As I began explaining the VM pamphlet, the inevitable question arose: "OMG, what am I going to eat!?"

When it came to my suggestion of chicken, the patient raised her hand in objection. "Oh no! We can't..." she protested. I was astounded as I questioned, 'What do you mean by 'we'?" Her answer, echoed by her mother and daughter, hit me like a ton of bricks: "Me, my mom, and my daughter—we can't eat poultry. Every time we do, we vomit."

The memory of my previous encounter rushed back with a pang of guilt and regret. How could I have doubted my patient' words all those years ago? It was a sobering reminder of the importance of listening to patients and taking their experiences seriously. After all, who was I to dismiss their lived realities? (At that time, I had yet to encounter the works of Aretaeus.)

While I never encountered another patient with a similar aversion to poultry, the lesson learned from those four souls resonated deeply.

Let's return to our topic. For a considerable period, extending beyond Aretaeus' era, migraine management centered around elimination diets. Recent literature, however, offers a more nuanced approach, incorporating diet suggestions and well-established trigger avoidance strategies. While these suggested diets still function as elimination diets in their own right—for instance, the ketogenic or modified Atkins diets, which have shown benefits, along with high omega-3 diets—they share a common emphasis on carbohydrate restriction. Additionally, low glycemic diets have demonstrated efficacy in migraine management.

Debates persist regarding the impact of low-sodium diets. Nevertheless, the challenges of water and salt metabolism, coupled with fluid retention in many patients, have been recognized since ancient times. Consequently, my inclination leans towards advocating for the limitation of salt intake, particularly during vulnerable periods such as seasonal transitions and heightened stress.

Vestibular Migraine Menu: Mastering the Art of Eating (Without the Spin)

> *Human beings, who are almost unique in having the ability*
> *to learn from the experience of others, are also remarkable for*
> *their apparent disinclination to do so.*
>
> – Douglas Adams

In today's world, navigating the ever-changing landscape of dietary advice can feel like an exhausting rollercoaster. From superfoods to gluten, antioxidants to carbs, the pendulum swings wildly between what's good and what's not. One moment, fat is deemed a killer, only to be hailed as a health hero the next. And don't even get started on the demonization of carbs or the flip-flopping stance on eggs – it's enough to make your head spin!

It's tempting to dismiss this dietary chaos as a modern invention, a symptom of our obsession with health and wellness. After all, diets seem to change as frequently as the weather: intermittent fasting, butter in morning coffee (not as gross as it sounds, but is it necessary?), the ongoing debate between vegetarians and vegans, and let's not forget Silicon Valley's jest-worthy "pesce-pescetarians." It's enough to make you question if sanity has left the building, right?

But here's the thing: the relationship between food and health is as old as the written word itself. Take ancient Greece, for example, where maintaining a balance of the body's four "humours"—black bile, yellow bile, phlegm (eww), and blood—was believed to be fundamental to good health. Dietary modifications were seen as the primary means to achieve this balance.

Food historian Francine Segan sheds light on ancient Greek dietary practices, revealing tales of athletes who thrived on protein-heavy diets reminiscent of today's Atkins diet. In her book, *The Philosopher's Kitchen*,[230] she uncovers documents from *The Deipnosophists* by Athenaeus, describing an

---

230 Bramen L., National Geographic News. Ancient Olympians Followed "Atkins" Diet, Scholar Says. *The History of Heath Food,* Smithsonianmag.com, October 13, 2009.

Olympic runner who dominated races while subsisting mainly on meat, which started a meat-only craze in public. Sounds familiar, doesn't it?

The intertwining of food and health extends far beyond what we could have imagined or wanted to accept. Yet if you're searching for dietary guidance to alleviate vertigo, you'll likely come up empty-handed in traditional research papers or books. Instead, turning to migraine-focused diet books may offer more insight.

We've been aware of potential migraine triggers since the time of Aretaeus,[231] but controversy has always been present in the field. Some well-known migraine triggers include chocolate, citrus fruits, dairy products, alcoholic beverages, coffee, caffeine, monosodium glutamate (MSG), histamine (found in alcohol, fermented foods, dairy products like yogurt, sauerkraut, dried fruits, shellfish, and smoked meats), tyramine-containing foods (such as aged cheese, tap beer, fermented or dried meats, soy sauce, miso, and red wine), nitrites (common in deli meats), aspartame, sucralose, and gluten, as noted in the literature.

While these triggers are statistically common, many more foods can trigger migraines. Remember the cautionary tale of Chicken à la Regret (page 179)

When discussing food intolerance or triggering foods, it's important to acknowledge the wisdom of Hippocrates. In his Phaedrus,[232] Plato wrote, "Hippocrates says that a physician should classify human beings according to how they react to a particular type of food. It is not sufficient to learn simply that cheese is a bad food … cheese does not harm all men alike; some can eat their fill of it without the slightest hurt; nay, those it agrees with are wonderfully strengthened thereby. Others come off badly. So the constitutions of these men differ… If cheese were bad for the human constitution without exception, it would have hurt all."

---

231 Hoffmann, J.; Recober, A. Migraine, and triggers: Post hoc ergo propter hoc? *Curr Pain Headache Rep.* 2013, 17, 370.

232 Jelinek, E., Pappas N., Hippocrates at Phaedrus 270 BC, *Pacific Philosophical Quarterly*. 09/2020, Volume 101, Issue 3.

While we're all humans, we are as unique as our fingerprints. Many physiological processes work tirelessly with individual tweaks. Food science, particularly concerning diets and their effects on us, resembles meteorological science in many ways. Both fields provide abundant data, but making on-the-spot predictions can be incredibly challenging.

Even the same food can elicit different effects on the same person at different times. A specific food trigger may depend on various factors, including the amount and timing of exposure.

Recall the puzzle metaphor, where all the pieces must fit together to create an episode? In each patient, the importance of these pieces may vary. You might be more sensitive to seasonal changes or exhaustion than to food; or conversely, you may be very sensitive to certain foods.

This quotation, attributed to Hippocrates, bears profound wisdom: "If someone wishes for good health, one must first ask oneself if he is ready to do away with the reasons for his illness. Only then is it possible to help him." While this may sound philosophical, it profoundly impacts our daily lives.

Imagine the typical breakfast rituals worldwide: fresh coffee or orange juice in some regions, black tea with feta, black olives, and bread in Turkey, or boiled rice with soy sauce in Southeast Asia. Breaking our ingrained habits can be challenging, but it's achievable. Moreover, once you identify your triggers, you'll find immense relief.

Following a dietary trigger, the severity of a vertigo episode can vary depending on factors like the amount and combination of triggers, timing of consumption, and other individual factors.

Certain ingredients, such as MSG, sucralose, or aspartame, may need to be consumed in high amounts to trigger a reaction, while caffeine can have a dual effect (withdrawal may also trigger an episode). While identifying triggers is crucial, more is needed due to the substantial variability among individuals and other contributing factors. In my practice, I've employed food diaries to aid patients in identifying triggering foods and beverages. These diaries serve as invaluable tools, not only pinpointing specific dietary triggers but also illuminating (surprisingly) habits that may provoke episodes.

Painting the Path to Vertigo

Mrs. H.N. was a 52-year-old retired university librarian grappling with a new and unwelcome challenge: recurring vertigo episodes that disrupted her once-serene life.

It all began six months prior, with a sudden vertigo episode accompanied by nausea and vomiting, followed by a heavy-headed sensation upon awakening. Initially sporadic, these episodes soon became distressingly frequent, occurring weekly or bi-weekly. Despite consulting several physicians, who offered varied diagnoses ranging from Meniere's disease to psychogenic vertigo and attempting different medications, her symptoms persisted, leaving her disheartened and somewhat sad.

"I don't want to lose my joy for life, but I'm exhausted," she confided.

Upon gathering her medical history, a crucial piece of the puzzle emerged: severe migraine headaches during menopause, which had subsided afterward. A glimmer of insight sparked within me. "Let's keep a diary," I suggested. "Record everything you eat, drink, and every activity, along with the timing of your vertigo episodes. Let's reconvene in three weeks."

Returning with her meticulously maintained diary, Mrs. H.N. shared a revelation: her wood- painting classes coincided precisely with her vertigo episodes. "Could it be?" she pondered aloud. "Is it possible?"

Following retirement, she had taken up painting as a hobby, relishing the camaraderie of fellow art enthusiasts. However, it appeared that the fumes from the paints were now triggering her vertigo episodes, which had evolved into vestibular migraines. Remarkably, she required no treatment; simply recognizing how her body reacted differently in the present compared to her past migraine episodes was sufficient.

While Mrs. H.N.'s story concludes on a positive note, the journey to identifying triggers is often fraught with challenges. Some triggers may have a delayed onset, complicating the cause-and-effect relationship. Moreover, patients frequently contend with multiple triggers that can exacerbate each other's effects, compounded by the complex compositions of many foods. Despite the arduous nature of the process, perseverance and determination ultimately prevail, offering hope for symptom control through trigger avoidance.

To Move or Not to Move?

No passion in the world is equal to the passion to alter someone else's draft.
— H. G. Wells

As the esteemed Aretaeus articulated, "Fatigue may be less harmful than bad digestion, but it is still harmful." While I concur that fatigue poses significant risks, particularly in our bustling modern era, I remain uncertain about Aretaeus' specific interpretation of "fatigue." However, his subsequent guidance sheds some light on this concept within the context of his time. "The patients have to go for a walk in the morning after bowel movement. However, they should not become short of breath and should be able to bear the effort. A walk after lunch is also very good. A drive may last a while, but not in the wind and not with the head in the sun. For Sirius is bad for the head." I imagine your reaction now, which must be similar to mine: "What! Really? Sirius..?"

Indeed, the mention of Sirius may seem ridiculous to most of us. Nevertheless, while there may always be a minute chance of elucidating its significance a couple of centuries later, our immediate concern should lie elsewhere.

Although fatigue and exhaustion could trigger any kind of migraine (headache, vestibular, or any other form), conversely, exercise helps, particularly in vestibular migraine patients.

The concept of modern Vestibular Rehabilitation is relatively recent in the history of vestibular disorders. The first paper about Vestibular Rehabilitation was written in December 1945 by Terence Cawthorne,[233] and 120 of his patients underwent labyrinthectomy with Meniere's disease diagnosis. Interestingly Cawthorne was shocked with the clinics of labyrinthectomy patients, and he reported, "The symptoms and signs that follow immediately upon an injury to the labyrinth are widespread and are often so terrifying in their intensity that observers unused to the ways of the labyrinth may find it difficult to believe that such a profound disturbance can be caused by injury to such a modest organ. "He vividly described his patients. "The overwhelming vertigo, the awful sickness, and the turbulent eye movements—all enhanced by the slightest movement of the head—combine to form a picture of helpless misery that has few parallels in the whole field of injury and disease."

Cawthorne emphasized the significant effect of vestibular disturbances on patients' overall health, stressing the primal importance of the sense of balance. He also underscored the psychological challenges, revealing that some patients equated their suffering to apocalyptic scenarios, with ensuing psychological disruptions potentially masking the root cause of their condition.

With his colleague Dr. Cooksey, Cawthorne created the head exercises, known by their names; Cawthorne-Cooksey exercises were used effectively until CRP maneuvers (Epley, Semont and their modifications), and they are probably still being used with some professionals somewhere.[234]

And how could we forget our old friend Aretaeus? What's truly remarkable (though perhaps not surprising anymore) is that Aretaeus even recommended chironomy, an exercise regimen close to dancing, for his vertigo patients.[235]

233 Terence C., Vestibular Injuries. *Proc R Soc Med.* 1946 Mar; 39(5): 270–273.

234 Cooksey F.S., Rehabilitation in Vestibular Injuries. *Proc R Soc Med.* 1946 Mar; 39(5): 273–278.

235 Koehler P.J., van de Wiel T.W.M., 2001.

In short, for vestibular migraine patients, staying active is critical, particularly during remission periods. Participate in activities such as walking, swimming, dancing, yoga, or Tai Chi—anything that keeps you moving. Avoiding inactivity is crucial for managing symptoms effectively.

Now I will tell you the furthest opposite stories of my two patients, Dr. A.S. and Mrs. M.K., related to motion.

Part 1. I Want To, But I CAN'T (Because It Makes Me Dizzy!)

It all began with a phone call from a university hospital in Eskisehir, three hours away. On the line was Dr. A.S., an anesthesiologist, a young and driven academic grappling with debilitating positional vertigo. We arranged a meeting, and she made the journey to MUNSI one afternoon.

"I didn't lie down for almost two years," she confessed, delving into the details of her battle with BPPV, which had struck her two years prior.

"Didn't you seek help from your OHNS or Neurology Department?" I inquired.

"Of course I did," she replied, "but they wanted me to lie down!"

"Well, that's the only way to determine if you have BPPV, which seems highly likely based on your symptoms, and to treat it with a CRP maneuver," I explained, trying to reassure her about the procedure's safety and efficacy.

After about half an hour of discussion to calm her nerves, I escorted her to the examination room. I performed a routine OHNS examination and then asked her to sit on the exam bed for a Dix-Hallpike maneuver. However, to my surprise, she hesitated for a moment and then abruptly jumped down.

"I can't," she said firmly. "It's impossible!"

I was taken aback. Here was a physician, an academic in the medical field, who comprehended the situation perfectly well. Yet her fear overshadowed everything else.

Despite her assurances to return when she felt better, we both knew deep down that it was unlikely. And indeed, she never did.

Part 2. I Would Love to, But I CAN'T (Because I Have Dance Class!)

Mrs. M.K. burst into my office like a whirlwind. ""Hi, my dear doctor, I've been eagerly awaiting this appointment," she exclaimed. "I'm dizzy; it's just awful, you know, of course, you know." Her words were punctuated with a delightful giggle. "I've been talking to my high school friends; none of them have vertigo and dizziness like mine. It's been going on for so long, maybe years. I even asked my pottery class friends, who said the same thing. Mine feels hopeless, my dear doctor," she lamented, followed by another giggle.

"You don't strike me as a dizzy person," I replied, returning her joyful smile. It was always uplifting to encounter a cheerful patient.

"Oh, it's terrible, believe me," she insisted, though I couldn't quite bring myself to believe it. We chatted a bit more before I escorted her to the examination room. There, my judgment was quickly corrected! She exhibited nystagmus visible to the naked eye, even without the aid of video goggles or any provocation.

"You certainly do have dizziness!" I exclaimed in astonishment. What a revelation!

Back in my office, she confirmed that she had been experiencing small vertigo episodes off and on for almost a couple of years, with some brief remissions in between. "My head has never felt clear for years, if I may say, "she added. Despite this, she remained vibrant and cheerful, refusing to let her condition dictate her everyday life. She continued attending meetings, hobby classes, and hitting the gym whenever possible. I found her resilience fascinating. After providing her with treatment, I referred her to my assistant for further guidance on diet, sleep, and lifestyle adjustments. It took some time to identify her triggers, but she was symptom-free ten weeks later.

Alright, let's get into a spicy topic: sex. Aretaeus didn't mince words, warning that "Sexual intercourse is bad for the head and nerves, an evil that one brings upon oneself." Pretty dire, right? But hold onto your hats, because Oliver Sacks chimed in with a bit of relief, mentioning that only a handful of his patients experienced worse symptoms after getting frisky. He said, "A few patients are unfortunate enough to experience migraines immediately following orgasm." Now, I haven't had any patients report post-romantic vertigo, but hey, maybe they were just too shy to spill the beans.

Allow me to put on my academic cap again; we understand that strong emotions have a potent effect in triggering classical migraine headaches, and undoubtedly the same holds for vestibular migraine patients. Oliver Sacks cites Liveing, highlighting that the intensity of the emotion matters more than its character, and Liveing further suggests that sudden rage is often the primary trigger. However, fright or panic can be equally potent, particularly in younger patients. Interestingly, Lieving says that moments of sudden joy, like unexpected good fortune, can also provoke migraines. Liveing even coined the term "arousal migraines" to describe these occurrences.

So, what's the game plan? Sometimes, it's about making significant changes; sometimes a lot, sometimes none at all. It's about accepting things as they are. The key lies in self-awareness for both patients and healthcare providers. By understanding themselves better, patients can take charge of their health journey, while physicians can guide them with tailored advice and support. It's a collaborative journey towards empowerment and well-being.

Unsurprisingly, Aretaeus recommends medication only after exploring alternative remedies for his patients. He suggests journeys from cold to warmer and wet to dryer regions are beneficial. For those living on the coast, he advocates bathing in cold seawater, swimming, and even rolling in the sand (don't worry, I'm rolling my eyes, too), emphasizing the therapeutic benefits of staying close to the sea. According to him, these treatments can target specific areas of the head while benefiting the entire head. As a last resort, if patients don't find relief through these methods, he advises using hellebore, a potent diuretic plant, to expel the disease.

While Aretaeus' suggestions may seem absurd or even quaint to modern sensibilities, I believe his patients genuinely benefited from them. Additionally, we now understand that seasonal and climatic factors can indeed trigger migraines, with some research indicating seasonal variations, specifically in vestibular migraine.

As you would expect, Oliver Sacks didn't drop back; he delved into how various weather conditions can impact migraines. He noted that any climatic extreme might trigger a migraine in susceptible individuals or at least be attributed to doing so. Storms and winds are classic examples, with some patients claiming a sort of meteorological clairvoyance, able to predict approaching weather patterns based on their migraine episodes. For instance, he wrote that one of his colleagues recounted childhood migraines that coincided with annual south-westerly storms in Zürich but were absent at other times. Others experience migraines during very hot or humid weather, with such conditions potentially inducing lethargy and prostration that predisposes them to migraines.

Over my years of working with patients, I've observed the same trend: spring and fall tend to be the riskiest seasons for vestibular migraine episodes, both in my patients and in myself. [236] [237] [238] [239] [240] [241] [242]

236 Brewerton, Timothy D; George, Mark S., A Study of the Seasonal Variation of Migraine *Headache*, 07/1990, Volume 30, Issue 8.

237 Li W., Bertisch S.M., Mostofsky E., Buettne C., Weather, ambient air pollution, and risk of migraine headache onset among patients with migraine. Environment international. 11/2019, Volume 132.

238 Pereira A.B., Almeida L.A.F., Pereira N.G., Seasonality of dizziness and vertigo in a tropical region. *Chronobiology International: The Journal of Biological and Medical Rhythm Research.* Volume 32, 2015, Issue 5.

239 Min Hee K., Chunhoo C., Epidemiology and Seasonal Variation of Ménière's Disease: Data from a Population-Based Study. *Audiology & neurotology.* 2020, Volume 25, Issue 4.

240 Meghji S., Murphy D., Nunney I., The seasonal variation of benign paroxysmal positional vertigo. *Otology & Neurotology.* 2017.

241 Jahn K., Kreuzpointner A., Pfefferkorn T., Zwergal A., Telling friend from foe in emergency vertigo and dizziness: does season and daytime of presentation help in the differential diagnosis? *Journal of Neurology.* Volume 267, pages 118–125 (2020).

242 Z Cao, X Zhao, Y Ju, M Chen, Y Wang. Seasonality and Cardio-Cerebrovascular Risk Factors for Benign Paroxysmal Positional Vertigo. *Frontiers in neurology,* 2020.

Blabbering about the Obvious: Eat Well, Sleep Well, and Relax

Almost all organisms eat and sleep, and all organisms have to deal with stress somehow. Still, when there is a specific condition, such as vestibular migraine, these mundane activities become of ultimate importance. The consistency of daily routines regarding eating, sleeping, exercise, and hydration directly impacts the frequency and severity of chronic or episodic vestibular migraine episodes.

Research by Woldeamanuel and Cowan[243] underscored the significance of maintaining consistent daily patterns. Their study revealed that irregularities in these routines were associated with increased migraine episodes. Similarly, a study conducted in Korea during the same year, utilizing a smartphone-based headache diary application, highlighted the strong correlations between stress (58%), sleep deprivation (55%), and fatigue (49%) with subsequent migraine headache episodes among 62 participants. While these studies specifically address migraine headaches, their implications extend seamlessly to vestibular migraine cases.

Neither skipping meals, intentional or unintentional fasting, nor gorging is suitable for people with a migrainous base. Taken together, consistent, high-quality sleep, regular healthy meals, and refraining from hunger are targeted behaviors for people grappling with migraines.

Mastering Vestibular Migraine: Empowering Behavioral Strategies

Managing vestibular migraine involves initiating behavioral changes similar to handling other forms of migraines. Even patients who meticulously track their sleep and diet may find adopting exercise routines or changing their food preferences challenging, as change is often met with resistance. Understanding behavior change's science and practical aspects can benefit patients and healthcare providers.

---

243 Woldeamanuel YW, Cowan RP. The impact of regular lifestyle behavior in migraine: a prevalence case-referent study. *J Neurol.* 2016;263(4):669–76.

Changing or establishing behaviors is a nuanced process that requires more than just education. It's crucial to involve patients in decision-making and proceed gradually to ensure sustainable progress. Given that stress is a potent trigger, coercing patients (or oneself) into behavior changes can exacerbate stress levels. Instead, identify behaviors directly linked to vertigo/dizziness, such as stress management or sleep patterns, and establish concrete, measurable goals. For example, setting specific dietary or relaxation targets is more effective than vague directives like "eat healthy" or "sleep well." Collaborate with patients to tailor recommendations and start with manageable relaxation techniques or meditation exercises. Providing actionable strategies yields better outcomes than merely stating the obvious, such as the detrimental effects of stress.

Another critical point is to track the progress. Checking what is going on in your or your patient's life, whether "the goal" is achieved or not, is critical to successful behavioral changes. Self-monitoring is vital to help you or your patient assess their daily activities and symptom connections. Discovering these relevancies by themselves is a powerful acceleration toward healing.[244], [245] By implementing these behavioral strategies and fostering a collaborative approach, we can empower patients to take control of their vestibular migraine management and enhance their overall well-being. Together we can navigate the journey towards mastering vestibular migraine, one step at a time.

Vestibular Migraine Diet: What's NOT on the Menu for Relief?

In considering what to eat or not to eat to alleviate vertigo symptoms, the focus shifts to dietary choices. While the list may seem restrictive initially, it serves a temporary purpose.

244 Park JW, Chu MK, Kim JM, Park SG, Cho SJ. Analysis of trigger factors in episodic migraineurs using smartphone headache diary applications. PloS One.. 2016;11(2):e0149577.

245 Rosenberg, L., Butler N., Seng, E K., Health Behaviors in Episodic Migraine: Why Behavior Change Matters. *Current pain and headache reports* 10/2018, Volume 22, Issue 10.

For individuals experiencing chronic vertigo or dizziness, adhering to this dietary regimen until symptoms subside can be beneficial. However, it's important to gradually reintroduce foods, using a food diary to monitor any potential triggers once symptoms have disappeared completely.

Similarly, following the dietary guidelines during episodes and gradually reintroducing foods afterward for those with episodic vertigo episodes can help manage symptoms effectively. Utilizing a food diary in this process is essential for identifying and managing triggers.

By approaching dietary changes systematically and with patience, individuals can gain better control over their vertigo symptoms and improve their overall well-being.

SALT (sodium): Avoid salt as much as possible; keep daily sodium intake under 2 grams. Don't forget that table salt is only one of the forms of sodium found in foods; if you are unaware, you may easily exceed the recommended daily dose of sodium; many processed and packaged foods also contain high levels of sodium. When shopping, check food labels for sodium content and opt for low-sodium or sodium-free options whenever possible.

1. Processed Foods: Processed foods are often high in sodium, making them potential triggers for vertigo symptoms. Cured or smoked meats, such as smoked salmon and bacon, as well as packaged or ready-to-eat foods, pickles, kimchi, and sauerkraut, are all examples of processed foods that may contain high levels of sodium. Be sure to read food labels carefully and choose no (or low)-sodium alternatives whenever available.

2. Prepared Sauces and Condiments: Many prepared sauces and condiments, including salad dressings, Worcestershire sauce, soy sauce, fish sauce, and similar products, are also high in sodium. When using these condiments, opt for low-sodium versions or consider making your own sauces using fresh ingredients to control sodium levels.

3. Beverages: Tomato and vegetable juices, as well as some fruit juices, may contain sodium unless labeled otherwise.

4. Snacks and Packaged Foods: Snacks like chips, crackers, cookies, and similar items are often loaded with sodium. Always check the labels of packaged snacks and choose low-sodium options when possible. Similarly, packaged spice blends usually contain salt, so consider making your own spice blends using salt-free herbs and spices.

5. Additionally, some over-the-counter supplements and medicines may contain high amounts of salt, so it's essential to read labels carefully and consult with a pharmacist if you're unsure.

CHEESES: Although most cheeses have high sodium content, therefore we can put them in the previous category, but especially aged cheeses can trigger migraines, so even if you are meticulously measuring your sodium intake and thinking to include a piece of aged cheese in your meal, be careful.

ARTIFICIAL SWEETENERS: Aspartame, a common artificial sweetener, is known to trigger migraines in some individuals. Be mindful of products containing aspartame and consider using natural sweeteners like honey or stevia instead.

YEAST AND FERMENTED PRODUCTS: I am sorry, but yeasted dough such as sourdough bread, donuts, and bagels must be abandoned (just for a short period, don't forget!) Similarly, vinegar and fermented products like pickles, sauerkraut, and kimchi are not suitable for individuals prone to vertigo.

CULTURED DAIRY PRODUCTS: Such as kefir and yogurt (although very rare, but you may be special) can be your trigger.

CHOCOLATE: It could be the hardest to avoid, but chocolates are one of the most common migraine triggers.

NUTS: Nuts and all types of nut butter. You should avoid all of them. Although peanuts are actually legumes, we can put them here too.

TOMATOES: Very (very) rare, but you must avoid fresh, juice, or paste forms at the beginning of an elimination diet.

(SOME) VEGETABLES: Very few vegetables like onions, beans, and corn should also be left out of your diet.

ALCOHOL: Avoid all kinds of alcohol in acute episodes.

CAFFEINE: Same as alcohol, avoid caffeine in acute episodes, be careful if you are in a chronic phase, and use as little caffeine as possible. Yet there is something different with caffeine than alcohol. Sometimes the abrupt withdrawal of caffeine may cause symptoms, too, so if you are an avid coffee or caffeinated beverage drinker, you should gradually leave it.

CITRUS FRUITS: Although not very common, some fruits may trigger migraines; therefore, bananas, berries, plums, papayas, passion fruits, figs, and avocados should be monitored as well.

SEA FOOD: Attention, fish lovers! It's best to be cautious with fish until you've entirely overcome your vertigo/dizziness. Once you're feeling more stable, you can gradually introduce them into your diet one by one. Fish is known for being one of the healthiest meats, particularly wild-caught varieties like salmon. But you have to be careful and be sure it is not triggering your symptoms. Wait until you are free from your symptoms, and start with some white-meat fish, such as cod. If you are ok, you can try another kind; if, for example, cod triggered your symptom, wait until you feel alright again, and then try some other fish, like flounder; you can continue as such.

I understand your concern. It may seem daunting to see a list of dietary restrictions, but I assure you, it's only temporary. These precautions are essential for managing vertigo symptoms effectively. However, it's crucial to remember that they are not permanent changes. As you begin to feel better and healthier, you can gradually reintroduce many foods back into your diet.

The key is patience and belief in yourself. You have the power to take control of your health and overcome these challenges. Remember, this journey is about you; with determination and perseverance, you can successfully navigate through it.

Vestibular Migraine Diet: What's on the Menu for Relief?

Why not begin with history for a bit of fun?

Hereps the green light for a menu around the year 200s AD from Aretaeus (please don't roll your eyes! I told you, he was a prodigy, and everybody followed what he said for almost one-thousand and seven-hundred years...) There is so much wisdom on that list, believe me....

- Bearded wheat washed with as much wine and honey as to taste well to the patients.

- Spice it up with caraway, coriander, aniseed, and celery. Mint and pennyroyal are the VIPs for promoting micturition and a touch of flatulence.

- Fresh meat, especially from roosters, wood pigeons, common pigeons (not-too-fat), and goats.

- Among fish, go for the ones from the rocks, and the best ones.

- Cooked veggies that promote micturition and defecation are your friends: mallow, blite, beet, asparagus, and cabbage. Lettuce is the superhero among raw veggies.

- Avoid roots like radish, rapeseed, and carrots—they might cause trouble.

- Exclude for thin, sweet, and slightly astringent white wine to keep things flowing.

- Desserts, except all kinds of dates, can be headache triggers.

- Figs and grapes in the fall are your seasonal go-to.

Indeed, Aretaeus' wisdom transcends time, offering insights that resonate even in our modern understanding of health. Trying roosters as a potential remedy is intriguing, albeit challenging in today's culinary landscape.

As for his observation on desserts and headaches, "All desserts, except all kinds of dates, cause headaches." Now we know reactive hypoglycemia, which happens when you eat simple sugars; it raises your blood sugar fast; consequently, insulin overproduces, causing a rapid decline in blood sugar, resulting in migraines. It's easy to explain now, but they knew then.

Let's transition back to the present day and explore what foods are beneficial for managing vertigo. First of all, moderation is crucial for maintaining a balanced diet and overall well-being. Your meals must be light and frequent; don't make yourself hungry, but don't become overly full.

Menu Makeover: Savoring What's on the Table for Vestibular Migraine

Here are some guidelines for making dietary choices to manage vertigo:

- Almost all kinds and categories of vegetables are safe except onions, some beans, and corn unless, you detect something special in your food diary. I didn't see a triggering vegetable in my patients, but, that doesn't mean it is impossible.

- Legumes. You may be surprised because beans and peanuts are not allowed, but there is a trick here: all beans are considered legumes, but all legumes are not beans. You can check the legume list on the internet, which is long.

- Grains. Rice! You can eat as much as you want safely. Oats, barley, rye, corn, quinoa are safe too. Although wheat is safe, yeasted dough products, such as sourdough bread, donuts, etc., may trigger migraines (it is rare, but you should know)

- Red meats. Fresh meats are safe, but processed meats should be avoided.

- Poultry is safe, except if you know you are uncomfortable with it.

- Apples, grapes, melons, and pears are safe options. However, exercise caution with all fruits, including berries, especially during episodes or if you have a chronic condition. For example, I once had a colleague/patient who experienced severe vertigo episodes triggered by strawberries and mushrooms.

By being mindful of these guidelines and paying attention to your body's response to different foods, you can effectively manage your vertigo symptoms and improve your overall well-being. Remember, everyone's triggers may vary, so it's essential to personalize your dietary choices based on your unique needs and experiences.

Quenching Your Thirst, Vertigo Style: What to Drink?

Water is your best bet—drink plenty of it, but don't overdo it! Water intoxication is a real concern, so aim for 30 to 35 mL per kilogram of body weight.

Fruit juices without added sodium are also safe options, as long as they don't contain any trigger fruits mentioned earlier.

Now, onto wine! While it's been celebrated for centuries, its health benefits are debated. (Well, even the word "debated" could be unnecessarily optimistic; new studies show there is *nothing good for you* in alcohol.)

During acute episodes, it's best to avoid all types of alcohol. However, if you're managing a chronic condition, you might experiment with tiny amounts of white wine and see how you feel. Be more cautious with red wine; there's always a chance of triggering an episode, even with a small glass of cabernet.

CHAPTER 11

NO, EVERYTHING IS NOT
A NAIL, ALTHOUGH...

Every Tool's a Hammer: Life Is What You Make It

– Adam Savage

CONCLUSION

Vertigo and dizziness significantly impact both the physical and psychological well-being of those affected. Dr. Hannelore Neuhaser, an esteemed epidemiologist and researcher at the Robert Koch Institute, has conducted influential studies on the incidence and prevalence of dizziness and vertigo.[246],[247]

---

246 Bigelow R.T., Semenov Y.R., Sascha du Lac, Hoffman H., J., Agrawal Y., Vestibular vertigo and comorbid cognitive and psychiatric impairment: the 2008 National Health Interview Survey.

247 Neuhauser H.K., The epidemiology of dizziness and vertigo. *Handbook of Clinical Neurology*, Vol. 137 (3rd series). *Neuro-Otology.* 2016, Elsevier.

According to Neuhaser, individuals experiencing vestibular vertigo and dizziness seek medical consultation (70%), take sick leave (41%), find their daily activities interrupted (40%), and may even avoid leaving the house (19%). Additionally, health-related quality of life is lower in those with dizziness and vertigo compared to those without.[248]

Analyzing data from the 2008 National Health Interview Survey balance module in the United States, Lin and Bhattacharyya discovered that 34% of dizzy respondents reported falls, while only 9% of non-dizzy adults reported falls. This stark contrast underscores the fear and reluctance of vertigo/dizziness patients to engage in daily activities and leave their homes.[249],[250], [251]

In summary, dizziness and vertigo rank among the most common complaints in medicine. Neuhauser estimates that as of 2016, 15–35% of the general population will experience vertigo or dizziness at some point, with prevalence potentially even higher depending on the study criteria.[252]

The 2008 National Health Interview Survey in the United States revealed alarming statistics: approximately 14.8% of adult Americans experienced dizziness within the past 12 months, equating to over 33 million people. The numbers among older adults aged 65 and above are even more concerning. About 19.6% (7 million) reported problems with dizziness or balance in the previous year, with 30% (10 million) reporting vertigo and a staggering 68% (24 million) experiencing balance issues.

These numbers are actually very upsetting and frightening. Several other studies confirm that about one out of three older adults report dizziness.

248 Neuhauser H.K., Radtke A., von Brevern M., Burden of dizziness and vertigo in the community. *Arch Int Med.* 168 (2008), pp. 2118-2124.

249 Roberts D.S., Lin H.W., Bhattacharyya N.,. Health care practice patterns for balance disorders in the elderly. *Laryngoscope.* 2013 Oct;123(10):2539-43.

250 HW Lin, N Bhattacharyya. Balance disorders in the elderly: epidemiology and functional impact. *Laryngoscope.* 2012.

251 Lin H.W., Bhattacharyya N., Impact of dizziness and obesity on the prevalence of falls and fall-related injuries. *Laryngoscope.* 2014.

252 Neuhauser H.K., (2016)

Since vertigo and dizziness are recurrent, annual prevalence must be higher than the incidence. Unfortunately, these high incidences and prevalence don't overlap the prevalence of the underlying disorders, most probably because of the underdiagnosing of especially vestibular migraine and its cohorts, such as BPPV and chronic dizziness.

Remarkably, rotational dizziness, often associated with or interpreted as vestibular vertigo, was reported in 20-30% of adults. When considering migraine incidence, studies have shown an age-adjusted prevalence of around 15.9% among all adults. Yet a 2018 article in *Brain and Behavior*[253] highlighted a stark contrast: while population prevalence studies reported rates between 2.6% and 21.7%, neurologists reported significantly higher rates between 27.6% and 48.6%. This disparity may stem from increasing knowledge and awareness of migraine's diverse manifestations.

Indeed, the clinical manifestations of "migraine" extend far beyond just headaches, and it's no surprise that these two statistics—migraines and vertigos—often intersect. Undiagnosed vestibular migraine stands as a significant contributor to the difficulty of many vertigo patients who wander about, seeking relief.

Regrettably, both migraine and the critical role of the vestibular system remain inadequately understood by both physicians and patients alike. This lack of understanding underscores the importance of raising awareness and improving education surrounding these conditions to ensure timely diagnosis and effective management.

FURTHERMORE

To see what is in front of one's nose needs a constant struggle.
– George Orwell

---

253 Yeh WZ, Blizzard L, Taylor BV., What is the actual prevalence of migraine? *Brain Behav.* 2018 Jun;8(6).

It's commonly believed that vertigo only arises as a prominent symptom of a peripheral vestibular disorder, typically associated with a significant disruption. However, a subtle decline in vestibular function is a more widespread yet lesser-known issue, particularly prevalent with aging, exacerbating balance problems in older adults. While we can't reverse the aging process, there's hope—we can mitigate its effects by raising awareness, implementing preventive measures, and engaging in balance rehabilitation to stave off falls and related complications.[254]

The elderly population endures with the gravest outcome of this oblivion, given that the presbystasis (the loss of vestibular and balance functions associated with aging) combined with vertiginous disorders inevitably cause balance problems, which are a strong predictor of falls in older age groups. [255], [256]

The elderly population bears the brunt of this oversight, as presbystasis, or age-related vestibular and balance function loss, alongside vertiginous disorders, inevitably lead to balance issues—a strong predictor of falls in this demographic. Meanwhile, the rapidly aging global population poses a significant public health challenge. Falls are already the leading cause of accidental death among those over 65, resulting in debilitating injuries, loss of independence, and increased reliance on assisted-living facilities, exerting a substantial toll on both individuals and healthcare systems.[257]

Hence, accurately diagnosing and effectively treating the underlying cause of dizziness/vertigo is paramount for patient well-being. While research supporting the hypothesis is still lacking, early identification of vestibular migraine and tailored lifestyle adjustments and treatments may yield positive outcomes and prevent dizziness and balance problems in older adults.

254 Fernández L., Breinbauer H.A., Delano, P.H., Vertigo and Dizziness in the Elderly. *Frontiers in neurology.* 2015, Volume 6.

255Felipe, Lilian, et al. Presbyvertigo as a cause of dizziness in elderly. *Pró-Fono Revista de Atualização Científica.* 20 (2008): 99-104.

256 Erica W., Luana C., Fall prevention in the elderly population. CMAJ. 2004 Sep 28; 171(7): 724.

257 Lin H.W., Bhattacharyya N., Balance disorders in the elderly: epidemiology and functional impact. *Laryngoscope.* 122 (2012), pp. 1858-1861.

Wrapping Up the Journey: Closing Remark

Many vertigo/dizziness patients require not just a diagnosis but comprehensive treatment. However, it's essential to go beyond merely labeling a patient's condition as "you have vertigo." Conditions like chronic subjective dizziness, phobic postural vertigo, subjective imbalance, and space-motion phobia, while sounding severe, essentially translate to "you have vertigo." Accurate diagnosis means understanding the patient's unique condition, a crucial first step toward effective intervention. Empowering patients with knowledge and fostering their understanding of the disorder are fundamental aspects of this process.